ABC of
Intensive Care

Second Edition

ABC series

An outstanding collection of resources – written by specialists for non-specialists

The *ABC* series contains a wealth of indispensable resources for GPs, GP registrars, junior doctors, doctors in training and all those in primary care

- **Now fully revised and updated**
- **Highly illustrated, informative and a practical source of knowledge**
- **An easy-to-use resource, covering the symptoms, investigations, treatment and management of conditions presenting in day-to-day practice and patient support**
- **Full colour photographs and illustrations aid diagnosis and patient understanding of a condition**

For more information on all books in the *ABC* series, including links to further information, references and links to the latest official guidelines, please visit:

www.abcbookseries.com

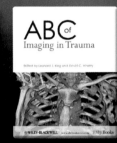
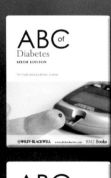
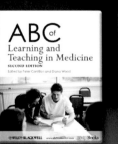
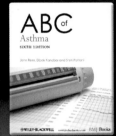
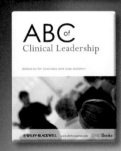
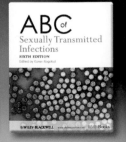

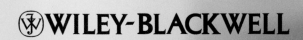

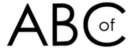

ABC of
Intensive Care

Second Edition

EDITED BY

Graham R. Nimmo

Consultant Physician in Intensive Care Medicine and Clinical Education
Western General Hospital, Edinburgh, UK

Mervyn Singer

Professor of Intensive Care Medicine
University College London, London, UK

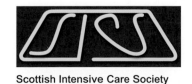

Scottish Intensive Care Society

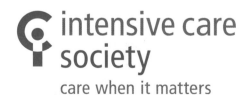

intensive care
society
care when it matters

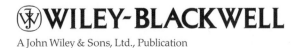

WILEY-BLACKWELL

A John Wiley & Sons, Ltd., Publication

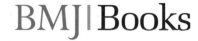

BMJ|Books

This edition first published 2011, © 2011 by Blackwell Publishing Ltd

BMJ Books is an imprint of BMJ Publishing Group Limited, used under licence by Blackwell Publishing which was acquired by John Wiley & Sons in February 2007. Blackwell's publishing programme has been merged with Wiley's global Scientific, Technical and Medical business to form Wiley-Blackwell.

Registered office: John Wiley & Sons, Ltd, The Atrium, Southern Gate, Chichester, West Sussex, PO19 8SQ, UK

Editorial offices: 9600 Garsington Road, Oxford, OX4 2DQ, UK
The Atrium, Southern Gate, Chichester, West Sussex, PO19 8SQ, UK
111 River Street, Hoboken, NJ 07030-5774, USA

For details of our global editorial offices, for customer services and for information about how to apply for permission to reuse the copyright material in this book please see our website at www.wiley.com/wiley-blackwell

Library of Congress Cataloging-in-Publication Data
ABC of intensive care / edited by Graham R. Nimmo, Mervyn Singer. – 2nd ed.
    p. ; cm.
  Includes bibliographical references and index.
  ISBN 978-1-4051-7803-7 (pbk. : alk. paper)
  1. Critical care medicine. I. Nimmo, Graham R. II. Singer, Mervyn.
  [DNLM: 1. Intensive Care – methods. 2. Critical Illness – therapy. WX 218]
  RC86.A23 2011
  616.02′8 – dc22

                                        2011008380

A catalogue record for this book is available from the British Library.
This book is published in the following electronic formats: ePDF 9781444345193; ePub 9781444345209; Mobi 9781444345216

Set in 9.25/12 Minion by Laserwords Private Limited, Chennai, India
Printed and bound in Malaysia by Vivar Printing Sdn Bhd

1   2011

Contents

Contributors

Sheila Adam
Head of Nursing, Surgery and Cancer Board, University College, London Hospitals, NHS Foundation Trust, London, UK

Peter J. D. Andrews
Consultant in Critical Care, Western General Hospital, Lothian University Hospitals Division; Professor, Centre for Clinical Brain Sciences, University of Edinburgh, UK

Anna Bachelor
Consultant in Anaesthesia and Intensive Care Medicine, Royal Victoria Infirmary, Newcastle-upon-Tyne, UK

Jonathan Ball
Consultant in Intensive Care, St. George's Hospital, London, UK

Simon Baudouin
Senior Lecturer in Intensive Care Medicine and Consultant in Intensive Care Medicine, Royal Victoria Infirmary, Newcastle, UK

Timothy W. Evans
Professor of Intensive Care Medicine and Consultant in Intensive Care Medicine, Royal Brompton Hospital, London, UK

Michael Gillies
Consultant Intensivist, Royal Infirmary of Edinburgh, Edinburgh, UK

James Haslam
Specialty Registrar in Intensive Care, St. George's Hospital, London, UK

Charles Hinds
Professor of Intensive Care Medicine, Barts and The London Queen Mary School of Medicine, London, UK

Chris Holland
Consultant in Adult Intensive Care; Lecturer, King's College Hospital, London, UK

Martin Hughes
Consultant in Anaesthesia and Intensive Care Medicine, Royal Infirmary, Glasgow, UK

Peter MacNaughton
Consultant in Intensive Care Medicine, Plymouth, UK

Marcia McDougall
Intensive Care Unit, Queen Margaret Hospital, Dunfermline, UK

Saif Al Musa
Clinical Research Fellow, St. George's Hospital, London, UK

Peter Nightingale
Consultant in Anaesthesia and Intensive Care, University Hospital of South Manchester, Manchester, UK

Graham R. Nimmo
Consultant Physician in Intensive Care Medicine and Clinical Education, Western General Hospital, Edinburgh, UK

Mandy Odell
Nurse Consultant, Critical Care, The Royal Berkshire NHS Foundation Trust, Reading, UK

Liam Plant
Consultant Renal Physician and Clinical Senior Lecturer in Nephrology, Department of Renal Medicine, Cork University Hospital, Cork, Ireland

Tony M. Rahman
Consultant Gastroenterologist and Intensive Care Physician, St. George's Hospital, London, UK

Andy Rhodes
Consultant in Intensive Care Medicine, St. George's Hospital, London, UK

Ben Shippey
Consultant in Anaesthesia and Critical Care Medicine, NHS Fife, Fife, Scotland

Alasdair Short
Consultant Intensive Care Physician, Broomfield Hospital, Chelmsford, UK

Mervyn Singer
Professor of Intensive Care Medicine, University College London, London, UK

Neil Soni

Consultant in Anaesthesia and Intensive Care Medicine, Chelsea and Westminster Hospital, London, UK

Tim Walsh

Consultant in Critical Care, Royal Infirmary of Edinburgh; Honorary Professor, University of Edinburgh, Edinburgh, UK

David Watson

Honorary Professor of Intensive Care Education, Barts and The London School of Medicine; Consultant in Intensive Care Medicine, Homerton University Hospital, London, UK

Julia Wendon

Consultant and Senior Lecturer, King's College Hospital, London, UK

Bob Winter

Consultant in Intensive Care Medicine, Queens Medical Centre, Nottingham, UK

Duncan Wyncoll

Consultant Intensivist, Guy's and St Thomas' Hospital, London, UK

Preface

Patients who require intensive care are usually the sickest patients in hospital. This is evidenced by their high mortality, and survivors may have persisting morbidities that may continue well after hospital discharge. They suffer from myriad diseases and can be referred from a diverse range of clinical settings: the emergency department, operating theatres, wards and even outpatient clinics. They present to intensive care when their diseases impinge on and impair the body's normal physiological processes, resulting in organ failures that may involve one or a combination of respiratory, cardiovascular, renal, neurological, gastrointestinal, hepatic, metabolic or other systems. Multiple trauma and sepsis are two of the commonest conditions that lead to critical illness. In order for intensive care to be most effective the unwell patient must be recognized, treated and referred early. Their subsequent management in intensive care needs to be scrupulous.

We provide updates on important advances in the understanding of the pathophysiology of critical illness, improvements in organ support and an insight into the human aspects of intensive care which are so important, including decision-making, communication and end-of-life care. The fundamentals of intensive care are covered in succinct, easy-to-read chapters written by experts in each individual area. The sum is a cohesive and contemporary introduction to the realm and speciality of intensive care.

As you read this book much of the mystery and awe which often surrounds intensive care will be dissipated and a real understanding of what can be achieved for the critically ill patient will emerge. Reading this book will enhance your clinical experience if you are a medical or nursing student approaching your first exposure to intensive care, a postgraduate medic or nurse on your first attachment, or an advanced practitioner in training. It will provide the medical or surgical specialist or general practitioners with a real insight to what is happening to your (our) patient when they require intensive care.

Graham R. Nimmo
Mervyn Singer

Foreword

Twelve years have elapsed since the publication of the highly successful first edition of the *ABC of Intensive Care*. Its publication, promoted by the UK Intensive Care Society, marked a crucial phase in the development of the specialty of Intensive Care Medicine (ICM). In the preceding 47 years since intubation and ventilation was first used in the treatment of respiratory failure, intensive care units (ICUs) had developed rather haphazardly across the world, led generally by local enthusiasts. Thereafter, from the 1970s, Intensive Care/Critical Care Societies in many countries across the globe have driven forward the organisation and development of ICUs, and created the specialty of ICM.

In our introduction to the first edition, Mervyn Singer and I declared that the specialty of ICM was 'coming of age'. Now, on reflection, this statement was perhaps a little optimistic at that time. Intensive Care Medicine in 1999 was largely practised within the walls of the ICU by a variety of clinicians from differing backgrounds with an interest in ICM; education and training programmes for future intensivists were still at a rudimentary level of development in many countries, and indeed the specialty was not even recognized as a distinct entity in most countries.

The intervening years have seen major advances notably in organisation and training, so that when this second edition appears on the bookshelves we shall truly be able to say that the specialty of ICM has come of age. Many doctors and nurses now choose ICM as their principal or sole specialty. Others in many specialties cannot function without regular interaction with and support from the critical care team. Increasingly, all doctors working in acute specialties receive basic training in ICM as part of their specialty training. Hospitals cannot function as emergency centres for medicine or surgery without the provision of an ICU and its attendant critical care team that provides care across the hospital.

Official recognition of our specialty was slow in coming, but in many countries across the globe this has now been achieved. The European Union has recognized ICM as a medical specialty, and in the United Kingdom an Intercollegiate Faculty of Intensive Care Medicine has been successfully established within the Royal College of Anaesthetists to supervise training, assessment and examination in the specialty, a development which 12 years ago was a distant dream.

Over these 12 years, there have been further developments in the understanding of the pathogenesis of sepsis and organ dysfunction, the technology of monitoring and organ function support, the importance of appropriate nutrition and, especially, in the area of early recognition and prompt treatment of the critically ill, ICU follow-up and post-ICU rehabilitation. The second edition will, hopefully, yield light on these and other important issues. While still dealing with individual organ system support as in the first edition, there are additional chapters on monitoring, sepsis, nutrition, sedation and outreach as well as broadening the chapter on 'withdrawal of treatment' to include the whole subject of 'end-of-life care'. Furthermore, important day-to-day issues of clinical decision-making and 'handovers' to maintain continuity of care are addressed.

The second edition of the *ABC*, like the first, will aim to balance scientific aspects of knowledge with practical guidelines for the management of critically ill patients. It will provide a useful introduction to ICM for those pursuing a career in an acute specialty, who require to be familiar with the scope, philosophy and practicalities of ICU management, and in particular for those doctors and nurses who are entering into a period of training in the ICU.

Ian S. Grant
Retired Consultant Intensivist
Western General Hospital, Edinburgh

CHAPTER 1

General Principles of Intensive Care Management

Anna Batchelor[1] and Peter Nightingale[2]

[1]Royal Victoria Infirmary, Newcastle-upon-Tyne, UK
[2]University Hospital of South Manchester, Manchester, UK

OVERVIEW

A critical care unit:

- is a specialized area concentrating care for the sickest patients in the hospital in one place
- is staffed by a multidisciplinary team of doctors, nurses, physiotherapists and dieticians, among others, who combine treatment with constant patient observation, monitoring and support
- has the equipment and medication required to provide multi-organ support
- needs to be physically close to operating theatres, emergency departments and radiology services
- is only the starting point for the patient. Patients and their families have needs beyond organ support: rehabilitation, both physical and psychological, should start during the time in critical care

---

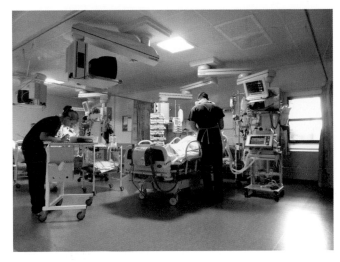

Figure 1.1 A critical care unit.

Places, people and patients

The term 'critical care' is used to encompass both intensive and high-dependency patient care. This type of care is normally delivered in units separate from general wards where most patients are nursed. Some specialist wards may have 'high-care' areas, although these are seldom equipped or staffed to an equivalent degree. Patients who require intensive care are usually managed initially in wards, operating theatres, radiology or endoscopy suites, or the emergency department. The staff in these areas need to promptly assess the patient, recognize the severity of their underlying illness, and initiate immediate life-saving management, while, at the same time, contacting the intensive care unit (ICU). An online tutorial covering this aspect of pre-ICU care can be found at: http://www.scottishintensivecare.org.uk/education/index.htm

ICUs and high dependency units (HDUs) (Figure 1.1) are typically centrally located within a hospital near to the emergency department, operating theatres and radiology department, but may be located in other specialist areas such as burns centres. This central

ABC of Intensive Care, Second Edition.
Edited by Graham R. Nimmo and Mervyn Singer.
© 2011 Blackwell Publishing Ltd. Published 2011 by Blackwell Publishing Ltd.

location is important to facilitate smooth patient transfer, e.g. to theatre for surgery or to the radiology department for imaging.

Nursing staff dedicated to the care of critically ill patients are trained specifically for this work; such patients are considered too ill to be cared for in a normal ward.

Intensive care is also called Level 3 (Figure 1.2) care, and is for patients requiring either invasive ventilation or the support of two or more failing organ systems.

High dependency care, also called Level 2 (Figure 1.3) care, is for patients needing non-invasive respiratory or other single organ failure support.

Treatment during a critical illness is not just about the patient. Caring for very sick patients is highly stressful to family, friends and carers, who all need support. Intensive care thus involves holistic support of the patient, family and friends, and also the referring staff.

The unit

Critical care is a relatively new specialty with its beginnings rooted in the polio epidemics of the 1950s in Denmark, where mortality rates were drastically reduced by tracheal intubation, manual ventilation (by teams of medical students) and the gathering together of patients in a single site. Subsequent to this, Bjørn Ibsen established what is considered the first proper ICU in Copenhagen in 1953.

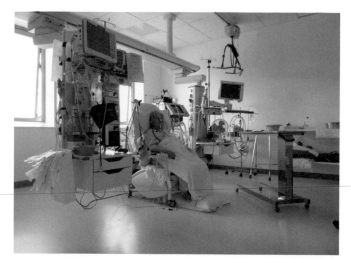

Figure 1.2 A Level 3 patient.

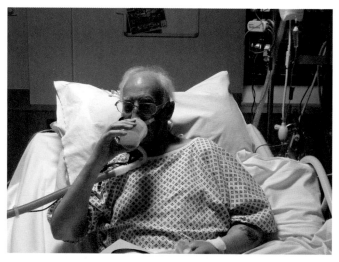

Figure 1.3 A Level 2 patient.

Initially, only patients requiring artificial ventilation were admitted to ICUs but the recognition that there were other patients needing a higher level of monitoring, observation and care has led to the development of HDUs or units that cater for both Level 2 and Level 3 patients.

Units vary in size; in the UK most have between six and 20 beds. Some operate solely as ICUs admitting the most seriously ill patients, whereas some are a mixture of intensive and high dependency care. In smaller hospitals the coronary care unit may be utilized for high-dependency patients with non-cardiac problems. In critical care it is common to have many patients in a large open area with curtains or screens to ensure patient privacy, and to have a few separate cubicles in which patients who are infected or are at increased risk of infection (e.g. neutropenic patients) can be isolated. Nowadays units are being built with proportionately more cubicles. However, although single cubicles enhance privacy, maintain patient dignity, and possibly contribute to a reduction in cross-infection hazards, it can be more difficult and isolating

for both the patient and the nurse caring for them. Studies have reported a higher incidence of preventable adverse events in patients isolated for infection control.

Only 2% of UK hospital beds are in critical care units compared with up to 25% in some US and German hospitals. It is not unusual for a critical care unit to be full. In this situation clinicians need to balance the needs of all the patients requiring higher level care. Difficult decisions may need to be taken. Patients are sometimes transferred between units because their care can be better delivered in a more specialist unit, for example after a head injury. Transfers not for the benefit of a patient sometimes have to occur because another patient is too ill to move and the unit is full. It is generally acknowledged that this is never an ideal situation. The transfer must be undertaken safely and with the consent of the patient, if possible, and of their family. The principles of medical ethics, beneficence, non-malificence, autonomy and justice can be used to guide practice.

There are many devices stationed by the bedside of a critically ill patient, including ventilators to support ventilatory function, machines to replace renal function (haemofiltration or haemodialysis), and a range of monitors, infusion and syringe pumps. Machines for blood gas analysis (including co-oximetry for carboxy- and met-haemoglobin) with the additional capability of measuring blood glucose, lactate, sodium, potassium, ionized calcium and total haemoglobin are usually sited within the ICU, thereby providing rapid access to these data.

A large amount of ancillary space is required for storage of equipment, including:

- gas cylinders with legal standards for storage
- disposable products
- a wide range of drugs
- laundry
- chairs for patients and visitors
- beds (for when patients are in chairs).

Clean and dirty utility areas and facilities for disposal of rubbish are also mandatory. Visitors should have a dedicated waiting area, preferably with comfortable chairs and television, and possibly with refreshment facilities. Quiet interview rooms for discussions with family members are essential. With office space, this all necessitates at least as much space again as that occupied by patients.

People

Critical care is delivered by a multidisciplinary team led by consultant intensivists. Intensivists are expert in the management of the critically ill patient. They have undertaken training over a wide range of medical areas including anaesthesia, general medicine and intensive care. They have the necessary skills to deliver and supervise the care given to patients with a wide range of organ dysfunctions and disease processes. They see acutely ill patients wherever they are located within the hospital, and not just within the ICU. They have skills in unit management, including the areas of finance, personnel and administration. They are educators at the bedside and in the classroom, not only to fellow doctors but to all members of the team. They show leadership, both clinical and managerial. They are the patient's advocate.

The referring clinician should visit the unit regularly and consult on their patient's management. However, while in the unit, the patients are managed hour by hour by the intensivist. Trainee doctors will also be present in the unit 24 hours a day, usually at a ratio of one for every eight beds.

Training in intensive care in the UK has been overseen by the Intercollegiate Board for Training in Intensive Care Medicine; however, this function has now been assumed by the Education and Training Committee of the recently formed Faculty of Intensive Care Medicine. Training is in a base specialty plus periods of intensive care and complementary specialty training. A curriculum for a training programme leading to the award of either a single Certificate of Completion of Training (CCT) or dual CCTs in Intensive Care Medicine and another specialty has been approved by the General Medical Council and the first trainees will be admitted in 2012.

Nurses working in critical care require the skills necessary to care for severely ill patients, including the use of the multiplicity of equipment needed to keep these patients alive. In the UK the nurse–patient ratio is usually 1:1 for intensive care and 1:2 for high dependency care, compared to the ratio of between 1:6 and 1:10 on a general ward. They may be assisted by one or more support workers.

Other members of the multidisciplinary team include physiotherapists, pharmacists, dieticians, microbiologists, ward clerks and data clerks. Important input comes from other groups including the radiology and pathology departments.

Patients

The patients in the ICU are the sickest in the hospital. They will have at least one and often several organ systems that are failing and needing support. About 40% of admissions are due to a surgical cause; many of these patients will be admitted immediately after major elective surgery. The remainder will have a medical diagnosis and be referred from either the emergency department, general wards, other departments or transferred from other hospitals.

In assessing a patient for potential admission it is important to consider if their situation is reversible and if they have potential for recovery. An ICU admission is unpleasant and expensive and should generally be reserved for patients who can recover; an obvious exception is for patients who are potential organ donors. It is often difficult to be sure which patients will survive so, inevitably, many patients die in the ICU. Depending on the type of unit, about 20% of ICU patients will not survive. Of those who die most will do so because of failure to respond to treatment or because, in the long term, they are unable to overcome the stress of their illness, often because of severe underlying comorbidities. In these cases interventional treatment is withdrawn, after detailed discussion with colleagues and family members.

Care of the critically ill patient requires a systematic approach to assessment and management. When requesting an admission the referring consultant or delegated senior member of the team should provide a comprehensive history, results of investigations, the diagnosis and plan of action. Referrals should be seen as soon as possible and the treatment plan agreed. On admission the appropriate monitoring and treatment is undertaken and physiological goals are set. These are reviewed frequently and changed as necessary depending on the results of investigations or response to interventions.

In addition to support for their failing organs, ICU patients need fundamental care including adequate nutrition, pressure area care, thrombo-embolic and stress ulcer prophylaxis, oral hygiene and psychological support. Much of this is provided by the nurse caring for the patient.

Many patients with infections will be admitted to intensive care so it is important to avoid transmitting infections between patients by the adoption of good hygiene techniques that are rigorously followed.

Relatives

Most units adopt an open visiting policy. The ICU is an alien and frightening environment so the presence of familiar faces and voices can be beneficial to patients. As critically ill patients may be limited in their ability to make or communicate decisions about their treatment, it is usual to ask relatives what choices the patient would likely have made had they been able to do so.

Problems after discharge

Many patients who survive an episode of critical illness have significant physical and/or psychological problems that may be life-long. Planning for rehabilitation now starts while the patient is still in the ICU. Merely surviving is not enough: it is crucial to ensure that the quality of life after intensive care is as good as possible within the bounds of any residual health problems.

Further reading

Critical Insight. The Intensive Care Society 2003. http://www.ics.ac.uk/patients_relatives/critical_insight.

Evolution of Intensive Care. The Intensive Care Society 2003. http://www.ics.ac.uk/intensive_care_professional/standards_and_guidelines/evolution_of_intensive_care_2003.

An Introductory Guide to Critical Care. The Intensive Care Society 2004. http://www.ics.ac.uk/education/a_guide_for_medical_students_and_junior_doctors.

Discharge from Intensive Care. The Intensive Care Society 2010. http://www.ics.ac.uk/patients_relatives/discharge_from.

General Information for Patients and Relatives. The Intensive Care Society 2010. http://www.ics.ac.uk/patients_relatives/patients_and_relatives.

Your stay in Intensive Care. The Intensive Care Society 2010. http://www.ics.ac.uk/patients_relatives/your_stay_in_intensive_care.

CHAPTER 2

Communication and Decision-Making in Intensive Care

Martin Hughes[1] *and Graham R. Nimmo*[2]

[1]Royal Infirmary, Glasgow, UK
[2]Western General Hospital, Edinburgh, UK

OVERVIEW

- Patients in intensive care are the sickest in the hospital
- The patient has often passed through several transitions of care prior to admission to the ICU: these include the community, wards and operating theatre
- There is often a high level of complexity
- Good-quality handover is pivotal; it improves patient safety and reduces error
- Good team leading and team-working with excellent liaison among the varied professional groups involved in patient care is vital
- The patient has usually had a diagnostic label attached to them before admission to intensive care but error is common and can lead to patient harm
- Methods are available to reduce diagnostic error

Introduction

Much of the activity in intensive care does not involve practical procedures or organ support. Thinking clearly, gathering, assessing and sharing information, weighing up situations and supporting others are all vital.

Particular areas of potential risk or uncertainty surround diagnosis and prognosis. These risks can be aggravated by poor handovers, inappropriate interruptions and unclear transfer of accountability. The critical care team needs to work both individually and collectively to optimize patient care and avoid error. This involves decision-making, task allocation, team working and situation awareness, all of which are underpinned by communication, cooperation and coordination.

These human factors (non-technical skills) have been labelled 'soft skills' in the literature. We would contend that they are actually hard skills: hard to quantify, hard to learn, hard to teach and hard to assess. This should not deflect from their importance in patient safety and quality of care: for example, diagnostic mistakes are one of the commonest causes of preventable error in clinical practice.

ABC of Intensive Care, Second Edition.
Edited by Graham R. Nimmo and Mervyn Singer.
© 2011 Blackwell Publishing Ltd. Published 2011 by Blackwell Publishing Ltd.

Handover

Handover of care is a bread-and-butter part of everyday clinical practice. Poor handover can be perilous thus good handover improves patient safety and reduces error. It should ensure continuity of care: comorbidities, diagnoses, clinical course, and individual therapeutic requirements are just some of the elements passed to incoming staff at a change of shift.

Clinical handovers take a variety of forms. The messages can be conveyed as written, verbal, printed, electronic or any combination of these. Verbal handover which affords the potential for discussion, although supported by the use of printed and handwritten information, appears to be the most effective at information transfer. All important events should be listed on a separate part of the patient's notes, so that vital clinical information is not lost because the ICU staff have changed several times. Clinical handover involves a transfer of professional responsibility as well as of information and clinical care, and should keep the patient's management plan moving forward. It can only be completed effectively if the clinician intimately knows the patients in his or her care.

Team-working and shared responsibility

Patients in intensive care have usually been referred by a specialty team and their management is conducted jointly between the core intensive care team, the referring team and the extended intensive care team (microbiology, pharmacy, physiotherapy, dietetics). The role of the intensivist is to coordinate this care and to apply expertise and knowledge of the context of critical illness to the standard management of less complicated conditions: the management of pulmonary embolism (PE) in a patient with intracerebral haemorrhage and acute respiratory distress syndrome (ARDS) is not the same as for a patient presenting with PE as an isolated diagnosis. The management of multiple organ failure, as opposed to single organ failure, requires the clinician to balance the burdens and benefits of proposed treatments, taking into account the competing demands of different organ systems. Fluid therapy in an underfilled patient may improve tissue perfusion, reduce inotrope or vasopressor requirements and increase urine output; however, if an unwanted consequence of intravascular filling is severe hypoxaemic respiratory failure then it will not be in the patient's interest.

Task allocation, planning and preparation, for example for admission or discharge, and juggling the needs of many patients (often in several geographical locations) requires good coordination and communication in addition to well-developed situation awareness throughout the team.

Interruptions

Interruptions occur during ward rounds, procedures, discussions with relatives or specialists, while checking drugs or equipment, or when prescribing and writing notes. They can take the form of face-to-face interaction, telephone calls or text messages, pagers, or alarms on monitors and equipment. They may be for relaying information, to refer patients, to discuss plans, to arrange treatment or investigations. Some are unnecessary and potentially unsafe, but others enhance patient care and safety by redirecting attention to more urgent clinical situations. Educational interventions could be used to reduce the detrimental effects of ill-timed interruptions and to promote effective redirectional interruptions.

Decision-making and diagnosis

There has been scant attention paid in the critical care literature to the importance of diagnosis. By a large margin, most consideration is given to methods of organ support, and how such support might be more effectively delivered. Patient safety initiatives have mainly focused upon a reduction in harm from interventions that facilitate or directly provide organ support (such as vascular catheter-related infection and ventilator-induced lung injury). The worth of this approach is well recognized. However, diagnostic error is the second biggest cause (after medication errors) of preventable error in medicine and may be associated with a proportionately higher morbidity than other types of medical error. Although the potential for diagnostic error is greatest in emergency medicine, general practice/family medicine and internal medicine, critical care clinicians are required to make, confirm or refute diagnoses in a large proportion of their patients. Even in critical care units with high doctor–patient ratios and advanced diagnostic facilities, post-mortem examinations suggest that up to 27% of patients have missed diagnoses that would have altered therapy had the findings been known pre-mortem.

How do clinicians think?

Contemporary psychology has divided cognitive reasoning into two basic processes, namely System 1 and System 2 (Figure 2.1). System 1 is rapid, intuitive, context sensitive and depends on pattern recognition. It allows experts to come to quick and often correct conclusions with a minimum of effort. System 2 reasoning is analytical and systematic. This system is mainly used to evaluate complex problems. During real-life clinical encounters the clinician usually toggles between the two systems; both are prone to error, or cognitive failure.

Cognitive failure

Despite its undoubted value, System 1 reasoning is more prone to error than System 2 reasoning, particularly for inexperienced clinicians. We are predisposed to a variety of flawed methods of

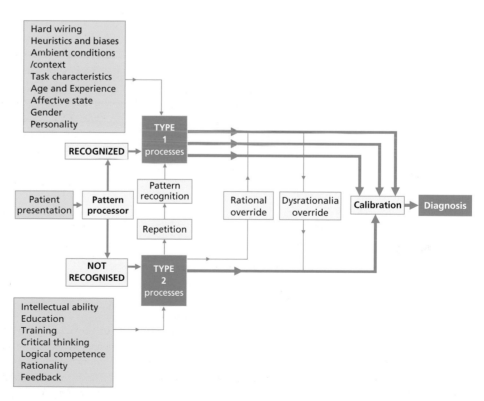

Figure 2.1 Putting it all together. We work using both System 1 and System 2 processes, all the time toggling back and forth between them with influences from all of the factors included in this schema. If we understand where we are situated cognitively we should be able to improve clinical decision-making (CDM) and patient management. *Source*: From Croskerry P. A Universal Model of Diagnostic Reasoning (2009). *Academic Medicine*, 84:1022–8. Reproduced with permission from Wolters Kluwer Health.

reasoning; there are at least 30 cognitive errors and biases. Most decision-makers and diagnosticians have made most of the errors at some time in their career.

Examples include the following:

- Anchoring – focusing on some important features of the initial presentation, and failing to modify this impression in the face of subsequent contradictory information.
- Confirmation bias – accepting confirmatory evidence to the initial diagnosis and ignoring or rejecting evidence refuting the diagnosis, even when the latter is more persuasive.
- Premature closure – 'when the diagnosis is made, the thinking stops'. Accepting a diagnosis before it has been fully verified. More information is needed.
- Search satisfying – calling off the search once something has been found. Comorbidities and other pathologies may be missed. The most common fracture missed in the emergency department is the second fracture. The information is there, but ignored. This may exacerbate anchoring and confirmation bias.
- Gambler's error – the four previous patients with chest pain have had acute coronary syndrome, so the fifth cannot also be acute coronary syndrome.
- Posterior probability error – confusion and agitation have been caused by alcohol withdrawal on the last four admissions, so this time it is also alcohol withdrawal and not, for example, hypoxia.
- Sutton's slip – when bank robber Willie Sutton was asked by a judge why he robbed banks, he said, 'Because that's where the money is'. Sutton's law is going for the obvious; Sutton's slip is when other possibilities are given inadequate consideration.
- Sunk costs – the more invested in a diagnosis (time, thought and personal reputation), the less likely the clinician is to consider another diagnosis.
- Investment bias – attaching more importance to information that we actively request or seek out than the information that was already available.

There has been a general reluctance to address cognitive errors, possibly because of a belief that these errors are simply part of the human condition – that we are programmed to think in these ways and there is nothing we can do about it. In order to address these errors, we have to accept that they exist, look for them and develop a reflective approach to diagnosis and clinical decision-making including metacognition – thinking about how we think.

Reducing cognitive errors

There are strategies available to reduce cognitive errors.

- Teach clinicians about cognitive errors, and make reflection on our reasoning skills and deficiencies (metacognition) routine. We should strive to be actively open-minded.
- Reduce reliance on memory with cognitive aids (mnemonics, computer-aided diagnosis). Make important information available in a clear and understandable format.
- Be familiar with critical data interpretation: what is the pre-test probability and how does the investigation alter the post-test odds?

In ICU we need to constantly question ourselves.

- In a complex clinical situation, what are the precise questions we are asking (e.g. what is the cause of respiratory failure?).
- List the differential diagnosis, with the evidence for and against each. Hypothesis generation is one of the earliest stages of diagnosis, and System 1 reasoning is often used to produce this first judgement. Central chest pain and cardiovascular instability are more likely to be caused by a myocardial infarction, but unless aortic dissection is contemplated, it is likely to be missed on those few occasions it presents. Differential diagnoses should be routinely considered (and listed) so that other less common or atypically presenting diseases processes are picked up.
- What new information (history, examination and investigation) is there and does it fit with the current diagnosis?
- Is there more than one diagnosis? A unifying diagnosis is what doctors usually search for. On average, this is more likely than multiple explanations.
- Is the available information correct and has it been personally checked? Examine the raw evidence for the diagnosis.
- Have I taken into account the potential biases of the clinician reporting information to me? It is sometimes difficult to challenge the established thinking of a colleague, but this is necessary if previous errors are not to be amplified. Diagnoses once made gain a momentum of their own as the patient moves through the system: they become *stickier*. Stop, examine the evidence and ask *'does this all fit together?'*
- Have I considered all the information given to me? We often remember the first and last part of a handover, and forget, or do not listen to, the middle.
- Am I using predominantly System 1 (heuristic, intuitive) or System 2 (systematic, analytical) processes, and is this method best for this diagnostic problem?
- Am I bored or depressed or annoyed by this patient and is that stopping me reassessing all the information?
- Is the direction and rate of progress as expected? If the patient is not improving on specific treatment reconsider the evidence
  - Is the diagnosis correct but advanced or aggressive disease is preventing improvement?
  - Is the diagnosis incomplete?
  - Is it one of several diagnoses?
  - Is it wrong?
  - Has a complication or a new diagnosis arisen?

What further investigations and treatments are needed, all things considered? Be clear on the reasons for your choice, and make a note of them where others can appraise your thoughts. Finally, re-evaluate – what have we missed or gotten wrong?

Final thought

Team-working, handover and decision-making pervade clinical practice. Multiple decisions are made in intensive care every day. Many of these pertain to institution of supportive measures such as ventilation or, in the improving patient, weaning of that support. However, the perfect application of multiple organ support counts for nothing if the underlying clinical condition(s) have not been diagnosed and if definitive *treatment* (as opposed to support) has not been instituted. We must constantly ask: 'Is this the correct diagnosis?'

Further reading

Blosser SA, Zimmerman HE, Staufer JL. Do autopsies of critically ill patients reveal important findings that were clinically undetected? *Crit Care Med* 1998; 26:1332–6.

Croskerry P. The importance of cognitive errors in diagnosis and strategies to minimize them. *Acad Med* 2003; 78:775–80.

Croskerry P. A Universal model of diagnostic reasoning. *Acad Med* 2009; 84:1022–8.

Graber M, Gordon R, Franklin N. Reducing diagnostic errors in medicine: what's the goal? *Acad Med* 2002; 77:981–92.

Nimmo GR, Mitchell C. An audit of interruptions in intensive care. *J Intensive Care Soc* 2008; 3:240–2.

Online tutorial

There is an online tutorial on this subject at http://www.scottish intensive-care.org.uk/education/index.htm. Click on the 'Induction tutorials' tab to find it.

CHAPTER 3

Monitoring

James Haslam[1], *Jonathan Ball*[1], *Andy Rhodes*[1] *and Peter MacNaughton*[2]

[1]St. George's Hospital, London, UK
[2]Consultant in Intensive Care Medicine, Plymouth, UK

OVERVIEW

- There is no substitute for regular clinical assessment
- Monitoring is not therapeutic. Timely and appropriate intervention based upon monitored variables *is* therapeutic
- Trends in measurements, especially responses to dynamic challenges, are usually far more informative than absolute values

---

Introduction

Intensive care involves the monitoring and support of multiple organ systems tailored to the individual patient. The environment in which this takes place is unique in the hospital setting for both the high staff to patient ratio and for the technology available. The most important and sophisticated monitoring modalities are the nurses and doctors caring for the patients. Monitoring in itself is not therapeutic and is only useful when changes are identified and acted upon in a timely and appropriate manner. In order to deliver optimal patient assessment, physiological variables are monitored to enable immediate/early recognition of deterioration and titration of organ supportive therapies. It is possible to classify the different types of monitoring used in intensive care by contrasting continuous with intermittent, or invasive with non-invasive. In practice, various monitoring modalities are often combined in portable integrated monitoring displays. This overview will utilize an organ systems-based approach to intensive care monitoring. Figure 3.1 shows a multimodality patient monitor.

Respiratory monitoring

The clinical practice of modern intensive care began with respiratory care units in the 1950s. Respiratory support remains an integral part of, and is often the principal reason for, intensive care. Various modes of monitoring are needed in order to gauge its necessity and efficacy.

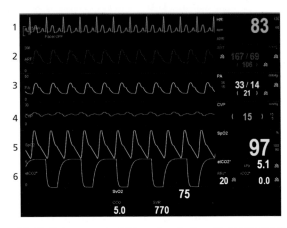

Figure 3.1 Multiple parameter ICU monitor display with continuous display of ECG (1), systemic arterial pressure (2), pulmonary artery pressure (3) central venous pressure (4), pulse oximetry (5), end tidal CO_2 (6), mixed venous oxygen saturation (SvO_2) continuous cardiac output (CCO) and systemic vascular resistance (SVR).

Respiratory function in patients receiving ventilatory support

All modern intensive care ventilators provide a wealth of respiratory function monitoring, not only to provide feedback data to the machine for safety and control purposes but also to provide continuous therapeutic monitoring of the fraction of inspired oxygen, respiratory rate (machine delivered, patient triggered and spontaneous), inspired and expired tidal volumes, minute ventilation, peak, plateau and end-expiratory pressures. In addition, pressure, flow and volume may be plotted continuously against time and displayed graphically. Many ventilators also provide extensive monitoring of lung mechanics, including compliance, resistance and intrinsic positive end-expiratory pressure (PEEP). The principal sensor involved is one or more forms of a differential pressure pneumotachograph, which continuously measures the pressure drop across a fixed or variable orifice, and integrates this against time to calculate flow and volume.

Pulse oximetry

Pulse oximetry enables continuous non-invasive measurement of arterial oxygen saturation. It utilizes transmission of red and infrared light through a pulsatile vascular bed, for example a finger or ear lobe. Absorption of light by oxyhaemoglobin and deoxyhaemoglobin is measured, and a percentage saturation is calculated. This is represented alongside a waveform of the pulse. In the majority of patients, pulse oximetry allows titration of inspired oxygen concentration, reducing the need for blood gas analysis. However, it may be unreliable in patients with poor peripheral perfusion.

Capnography

Capnography is the continuous monitoring of the partial pressure of CO_2 in inspired and expired gas. There are two main designs for such monitors, 'in line' and 'side stream'. They both utilize infrared absorption to measure the partial pressure generating a waveform of CO_2 over time. This not only provides a measurement of alveolar CO_2 which closely matches arterial CO_2 if the patient has normal lungs, but also valuable information regarding respiratory rate, respiratory mechanics, cardiac output and global metabolism. It can also provide an alert to emergencies such as oesophageal intubation, disconnection from ventilatory support and pulmonary embolism. In patients with significant pulmonary pathology there is often a poor relationship between alveolar CO_2 and arterial CO_2.

Blood gas analysis

In addition to measuring the partial pressures of oxygen and CO_2, blood gas analysers also measure or derive acid–base status (pH, bicarbonate, base excess, lactate), various electrolytes (including Na^+, K^+, Cl^-, Ca^{2+}), haemoglobin, glucose and lactate concentrations. Co-oximeters can also measure other haemoglobin fractions, for example carboxy-haemoglobin, met-haemoglobin.

Cardiovascular monitoring

Perhaps the most familiar monitoring in any hospital environment is that used in the assessment of the cardiovascular system.

Electrocardiogram

Cardiac electrical activity is monitored to identify heart rate, axis, rhythm and the presence of ischaemia or infarction, plus other abnormalities ranging from pericarditis to electrolyte disturbances. Continuous monitoring with three or five leads is standard practice principally for monitoring rate and rhythm. A full 12-lead electrocardiogram (ECG) is usually reserved for intermittent, but more detailed diagnostic use.

Non-invasive blood pressure measurement

This utilizes oscillotonometry to measure systolic, mean and diastolic arterial blood pressures. A cuff is inflated above systolic blood pressure to occlude blood flow. The return of blood flow, as the cuff deflates, causes oscillations in cuff pressure which are detected by a transducer that converts this mechanical pressure into an electrical signal. The onset of rapidly increasing oscillations corresponds to systolic pressure, maximum oscillation to mean arterial blood pressure and the onset of rapidly decreasing oscillations to diastolic pressure. Profound circulatory shock and arrhythmias can result in inaccuracies in pressure measurement.

Invasive arterial pressure measurement

Arterial pressures can be monitored continuously, on a beat-to-beat basis, using invasive arterial cannulation. Commonly, a fluid column is connected via a diaphragm to a transducer whose signal is amplified, undergoes analogue to digital conversion and is then displayed in real time. The system must be calibrated and zeroed and poor traces (resulting in either over- or under-'damped' signals) corrected to improve accuracy. In addition to arterial pressures, other information may be derived from the shape of the arterial pressure waveform including abnormalities of the aortic valve, the likelihood of volume responsiveness and the stroke volume (see below).

Arterial cannulation also allows for intermittent arterial blood sampling. The radial artery or dorsalis pedis arteries are commonly used though in the shocked patient the femoral artery may be particularly useful.

Central venous pressure

In a manner similar to invasive arterial pressure monitoring, the central venous pressure (CVP) may also be monitored via a central venous catheter whose tip is usually sited in the superior vena cava via the internal jugular or subclavian vein. To obtain accurate and reproducible measurements, it is essential that the transducer is levelled correctly to the estimated position of the right atrium (mid-axillary line: phlebostatic axis). The CVP provides an estimate of right ventricular end-diastolic pressure (RVEDP), which is a surrogate of right ventricular pre-load. However, a static 'resting' measurement of CVP is neither a good indicator of intravascular volume status nor the likely response to a volume challenge as it is affected both by changes in ventricular and vascular tree compliance and by intrathoracic pressure. Consequently, it is influenced to an unpredictable extent by positive pressure ventilation.

The central venous waveform can provide information about cardiac rhythm and will demonstrate significant tricuspid regurgitation. The variation in CVP with inspiration (the 'respiratory swing') correlates with changes in intrathoracic pressure and the work of breathing, although this is crucially affected by the size of the tidal volume. Central venous oxygen saturation is a surrogate (though not as accurate) marker of mixed venous (i.e. pulmonary artery) saturation, which indicates the global oxygen supply–demand balance. This is a useful marker of the adequacy of the cardiorespiratory system to deliver sufficient oxygen to the body as a whole, and is a target used to determine the success of resuscitation.

Cardiac output

Blood pressure is also a poor marker of the adequacy of tissue and organ perfusion. Cardiac output, or more specifically oxygen delivery (cardiac output × oxygen carried per unit volume of blood) is a far better measure and is often a principal target of goal-directed cardiovascular supportive therapies. It can be measured using a variety of techniques.

Pulmonary artery catheter

Here, the pulmonary artery is catheterized using a balloon-tipped, flow-directed catheter inserted via a sheath into a central vein. The balloon acts as a 'sail', 'floating' the catheter in the direction of blood flow until the tip comes to rest in a branch of the pulmonary artery. The catheter also has a lumen to inflate/deflate the balloon and a proximal lumen in the right atrium, to measure CVP. There may be other lumens to enable drug administration (including directly into the pulmonary circulation) and there may be connections to a thermistor, oximeter and/or pacing wire. Pulmonary artery catheters (PACs) can provide a host of information including gas tensions, oxygen saturations and pressure measurements from various parts of the right heart circulation. Key measurements include pulmonary artery pressure, pulmonary artery occlusion ('wedge') pressure (a proxy marker of left atrial pressure, measured by transducing the pressure from the distal lumen with the balloon inflated to occlude the pulmonary artery branch), right ventricular end-diastolic volume, ejection fraction and cardiac output using a temperature based, dilutional (thermodilution) technique (see below). Other data may also be derived including stroke volume, systemic and pulmonary vascular resistance. The use of PACs has fallen dramatically over recent years with the advent of less invasive devices. In patients with more complex circulatory pathology (e.g. pulmonary hypertension and systemic hypotension) the information gained from the PAC may still be very useful in titrating therapy.

Dilution techniques

Thermal dilution methods involve the use of either boluses of cold injectate or a thermal filament within the catheter emitting pulses of heat. Temperature change of blood, measured via a thermistor located at the tip of the catheter sitting in the pulmonary artery (or a proximal systemic artery), is plotted against time generating a curve, the area under which is inversely proportional to cardiac output. Alternatively, lithium can be used by injection of a known quantity into a large vein with the concentration being subsequently measured via a lithium-sensitive electrode in blood sampled from an arterial cannula. The lithium electrode is affected by concurrent administration of muscle relaxants. All dilution techniques are affected by tricuspid regurgitation.

Arterial pulse contour analysis

The systemic arterial pressure waveform can be analysed on a beat-to-beat basis in order to estimate cardiac output. The accuracy of this method is enhanced by periodic calibration using either thermal or lithium dilution. Caution is required in patients on vasopressors as these have been shown to affect the pulse waveform in peripheral arteries.

Oesophageal Doppler

An insulated ultrasound probe is inserted via the mouth or nose into the distal oesophagus, which lies parallel to the descending thoracic aorta. The velocity of descending aortic blood flow is measured utilizing the Doppler effect. This information, coupled with an estimate of aortic diameter based upon age, sex, height and weight, is then used to estimate beat-by-beat stroke volume and hence cardiac output. The waveform shape provides additional information on left ventricular preload, afterload and contractility.

Care must be taken if the patient has known pharyngo-oesophageal pathology. The cardiac output value may be affected by epidural anaesthesia, which increases blood flow to the lower body, or by moderate-to-severe aortic regurgitation.

Echocardiography

There are a variety of echocardiographic techniques that can estimate stroke volume and hence cardiac output from either transcutaneous or transoesophageal approaches. A wealth of additional information regarding cardiac function and structure may also be gained, including intravascular volume status, wall motion abnormalities, pericardial effusions and valve abnormalities. The major disadvantages of this technique are the skill required to make the measurements accurately and the intermittent nature of the monitoring.

Local and regional methods to assess perfusion

With advances in vascular imaging, bedside Doppler imaging of individual arteries is now possible. The most widely used is transcranial Doppler of the circle of Willis and the vertebro-basilar system (see also brain monitoring below), which is available as a continuous technique. Intermittent monitoring of hepatic and renal arterial flow is also possible.

Near-infrared spectroscopy (NIRS) is another light absorption method analogous to pulse oximetry that monitors oxy-haemoglobin levels within the microvasculature. It can be used as a continuous method to assess tissue (in particular, muscle and brain) oxygenation and perfusion. Dynamic testing utilizing an externally applied occlusion manoeuvre provides additional useful information on local delivery and utilization of oxygen. Some more sophisticated NIRS devices are able to monitor the redox status of cytochrome aa_3, the terminal electron acceptor of the mitochondrial electron transport chain. This is a superior indicator of the adequacy of tissue oxygenation but can only follow trends.

Renal monitoring

Routine indicators of kidney function used in critically ill patients are no different from the general ward patient and include urine output, serum and urine urea, creatinine, osmolality and electrolytes. Newer biomarkers such as neutrophil gelatinase-associated lipocalin (NGAL) and cystatin C may prove more sensitive markers of renal dysfunction than urea and creatinine, but require further validation.

Gastrointestinal, hepatic and intra-abdominal monitoring

Gastrointestinal monitoring is principally clinical. Although methods do exist for more detailed monitoring, such as gastric mucosal pH measurement, these are rarely employed outside of research investigations.

Relatively non-invasive hepatocyte function monitoring can be performed by injection of indocyanine green (ICG) into a major vein while monitoring blood levels utilizing an adapted transcutaneous spectrophotometer, again analogous to pulse oximetry. ICG clearance is dependent upon hepatic perfusion and hepatocyte uptake and excretion into bile.

Intermittent and continuous technologies exist to measure intra-abdominal pressure. It has been increasingly recognized that intra-abdominal hypertension and the abdominal compartment syndrome are common and a serious complication in a wide variety of critically ill patients. The commonest measurement method employs the urethral catheter, to which some form of pressure measuring apparatus is connected. A small volume of sterile water is instilled into the urinary bladder prior to each measurement. Internationally agreed guidelines on use have recently been published.

Brain monitoring

A number of complimentary modalities exist to monitor global brain perfusion and function. Intracranial pressure (ICP) can be measured continuously from a microtransducer inserted into the brain parenchyma or by connecting a fluid-filled pressure transducer to an external ventricular drain. Global haemodynamic and brain-specific therapies are targeted to maintain an adequate cerebral perfusion pressure (mean arterial pressure – ICP), usually aiming for over 60 mmHg. Transcranial Doppler can be used to assess regional perfusion (see above). The oxygen saturation in the jugular bulb may also be monitored following retrograde cannulation of the internal jugular vein by an oximetry catheter and can be used to assess global brain oxygen supply–demand balance and lactate levels as markers of aerobic and anaerobic metabolism. Continuous bifrontal, or bitemporal, electroencephalography can be very useful, either as raw or, more frequently, processed data, in assessing depth of coma and the detection and management of subclinical seizure activity.

Further reading

Anderson CT, Breen PH. Carbon dioxide kinetics and capnography during critical care. *Crit Care* 2000; 4: 207–15.

Cheatham M, Malbrain M, Kirkpatrick A, *et al.* Results from the International Conference of Experts on Intra-abdominal Hypertension and Abdominal Compartment Syndrome. II. Recommendations. *Intensive Care Med* 2007; 33: 951–62.

Creteur J. Muscle StO2 in critically ill patients. *Curr Opin Crit Care* 2008; 14: 361–6.

Faybik P, Hetz H. Plasma disappearance rate of indocyanine green in liver dysfunction. *Transplant Proc* 2006; 38: 801–2.

Lucangelo U, Bernabe F, Blanch L. Respiratory mechanics derived from signals in the ventilator circuit. *Respir Care* 2005; 50: 55–65.

Online tutorial

There is an online tutorial on this subject at http://www.scottish intensive-care.org.uk/education/index.htm. Click on the 'Induction tutorials' tab to find it.

CHAPTER 4

Sedation

Tim Walsh

Royal Infirmary of Edinburgh and University of Edinburgh, Edinburgh, UK

OVERVIEW

- Providing adequate sedation and analgesia are essential to minimize anxiety and pain, and to enable tolerance of essential interventions such as mechanical ventilation, physiotherapy and therapeutic procedures
- Sedation and analgesia are usually provided by continuous infusions of hypnotic and analgesic drugs
- Each patient should have an optimum sedation state defined and reviewed regularly, with clinical sedation scores and protocols used to ensure this target is achieved.
- Both under- and oversedation result in worse patient outcomes
- Delirium is very common in critically ill patients
- Patients should be screened regularly for the presence of delirium and management adjusted to minimize its duration

What is sedation?

Sedation is the reduction of conscious level by administration of drugs, either intermittently or by continuous infusion. Sedation requirements should be considered in conjunction with the need for pain relief, because many patients requiring intensive care may also have pain (e.g. from recent surgery) or will be undergoing treatments/procedures that cause pain or discomfort (e.g. physiotherapy or wound dressing). Most patients who require mechanical ventilation via an endotracheal tube will require sedation.

Why do patients in intensive care require sedation?

Some common reasons for administering sedation and analgesia in intensive care are shown in Table 4.1. The choice of drugs and the balance between sedation and analgesia depend on the requirements of the individual patient.

ABC of Intensive Care, Second Edition.
Edited by Graham R. Nimmo and Mervyn Singer.
© 2011 Blackwell Publishing Ltd. Published 2011 by Blackwell Publishing Ltd.

Drugs used to sedate patients in intensive care

Commonly used sedative drugs and some of their important properties are listed in Table 4.2. These agents account for a high proportion of total drug costs in intensive care. Choice of drug depends on the risk–benefit balance for an individual patient, but also on individual unit policies and protocols, and a consideration of cost, which can vary markedly. The pharmacokinetics and pharmacodynamics of sedative drugs are often unpredictable in critically ill patients because of increased sensitivity to the agents (e.g. due to encephalopathy), altered metabolism resulting from organ failure (especially renal and hepatic) and drug interactions altering metabolism. Regular review of the choice and dose of sedative agent is therefore important.

Optimum sedation

There is no single level or prescription for sedation that is suitable for all patients. Individual patient requirements frequently change as the underlying disease processes and therapeutic requirements evolve. There is thus a need for regular re-evaluation. For example, early on in critical illness requirements may be high because patients need to tolerate an orotracheal tube and controlled mechanical ventilation. Analgesic requirements may be high (e.g. post-operatively or following multiple trauma) while the need for anxiolysis may be a major consideration. In contrast, a patient who has been in intensive care for a prolonged period of time and with a tracheostomy *in situ* may not require any treatment except for boluses during uncomfortable procedures. In patients with critical oxygenation or with significantly raised intracranial pressure, sedation is pivotal and muscle relaxants may be used in conjunction with sedative and analgesic drugs. Sedation holds are inappropriate in these patients.

Optimum sedation is therefore the most appropriate level of sedation for an individual at the time of assessment. It is important to avoid both inadequate and excessive sedation because these can result in complications that worsen patient outcomes (Table 4.3). Doses of sedation should be sufficient for indications listed in Table 4.1, but should not cause an excessive and unnecessary reduction in conscious level. This balance is best achieved by establishing clear sedation management strategies. This often needs

Table 4.1 Reasons for sedating patients and providing analgesia in the intensive care unit.

Reason	Main requirement	Commonly used drugs	Comment
Anxiety	Hypnosis and anxiolysis	Benzodiazepines (midazolam; lorazepam) Propofol	Anxiety can result from fear concerning the underlying condition, ongoing treatments (especially invasive procedures such as mechanical ventilation) and difficulty in communicating
Amnesia	Hypnotics with amnesic properties	Benzodiazepines Propofol	Inducing amnesia is controversial. Prolonged amnesia during ICU care is associated with a higher prevalence of long term psychological problems (especially post-traumatic stress disorder)
Endotracheal intubation	Tolerance of endotracheal tube (decreased cough and gag) reflexes)	Opioids (alfentanil; fentanyl; morphine) Sedatives (propofol; benzodiazepines)	Endotracheal tube tolerance is highly variable. Older patients (especially those with COPD) often tolerate the tube with little sedation, but individual assessment is needed
Mechanical ventilation	To decrease respiratory drive; permit optimum synchronization with ventilator	Opioids and sedatives	Modern ventilators have modes that allow good synchrony with individual patient breathing patterns. Patient-ventilator dyssynchrony requires careful optimization of ventilator settings and sedation
Wound pain or other painful conditions	Analgesia	Opioids. Some regional anaesthetic techniques are valuable, especially after surgery or trauma	Ensuring adequate analgesia in patients with reduced conscious level from underlying condition or sedation is essential
Physiotherapy	Analgesia, anxiolysis, and anti-nociception	Opioids and hypnotics. Often best given as boluses during treatments	Physiotherapy, especially chest physiotherapy, is highly stimulating and can cause intense sympathetic activation via stimulation of intrapulmonary receptors.
Drug withdrawal	Control of withdrawal syndromes	Alcohol (benzodiazepines) Nicotine (nicotine patches) Heroin/methadone (opioids) Clonidine	Drug withdrawal syndromes are common in patients requiring critical care. Specific treatment should be considered particularly for patients not receiving sedation for other reasons

*COPD, chronic obstructive pulmonary disease.

Table 4.2 Consequences of inadequate and excessive sedation.

Consequences of inadequate sedation	Agitation Accidental extubation, removal of lines and tubes Lack of synchronization with mechanical ventilation Hypertension; tachycardia Myocardial ischaemia Increased oxygen demands
Consequences of excessive sedation	Hypotension and increased vasopressor use Delayed recovery of consciousness, delayed weaning from mechanical ventilation Ventilator associated pneumonia Prolonged intensive care stay Immunosuppression

significant education of staff and regular audit cycles to ensure continued implementation.

Practical aspects of managing sedation

Measuring sedation state

A clinical sedation scale that uses patient responses to simple stimuli should be used at regular intervals to categorize a patient's level of sedation. Many sedation scales exist; however, the Richmond Agitation–Sedation Scale (RASS) is the most widely validated and has high reproducibility when performed by nursing staff (Figure 4.1). Assessment starts with observation and progresses through non-physical and then physical stimulation if patients fail to respond. The Glasgow Coma Scale was designed to assess non-sedated patients with brain injury and is not suited to sedation assessment for patients without brain injury. Frequency of clinical sedation scoring by nursing staff is usually determined by individual unit protocols but, in general, should be carried out every 1–2 hours, especially when the patient's requirements are varying.

Sedation protocols

Intensive care units should have a protocol that summarizes the agreed approach to managing sedation in the local patient population. Protocols usually define the type and frequency of clinical sedation scoring that nursing staff should carry out. A target sedation state should be agreed at regular intervals with medical staff, based on individual patient needs. Effective protocols then empower nursing staff to adjust doses of sedative and analgesic drugs in response to clinical sedation scores to achieve the target sedation level. For many critically ill patients, a target of a responsive, 'lightly sedated' patient can be set without formal medical review. Maintaining this level of sedation can potentially shorten

Table 4.3 Some commonly used agents used for sedation in intensive care.

Drug	Main Effects	Duration of action (after dose change or stopping infusion)	Side effects	Potential for accumulation	Relative cost
Midazolam	Hypnosis amnesia; anxiolysis	Short (<1 h)	Mild hypotension Respiratory depression	Can accumulate with multiple dosing or continuous infusion, especially in presence of renal and hepatic dysfunction. Active metabolite (hydroxymidazolam)	Low
Lorazepam	Hypnosis; amnesia; anxiolysis	Intermediate (2–6 h)	Respiratory depression	Potential for accumulation, especially in renal or hepatic failure. No active metabolite	Low
Propofol	Hypnosis; anxiolysis	Short (<1 h)	Hypotension Respiratory depression Hyperlipidaemia and metabolic acidosis with high doses	Low probability of accumulation. No active metabolites.	Intermediate
Central α_2-agonists (Clonidine; dexmedetomidine*)	Hypnosis	Short (<1 h)	Bradycardia Hypotension	Low probability of accumulation	Intermediate/High

*Dexmedetomidine is not yet licensed for use in all countries (notably European countries), and is only licensed for short-term use in intensive care (<24 h).

intensive care stay and limit the complications of excessive sedation. Simple checklists can define those patients for whom medical review is not required before lightening of sedation (Box 4.1). In addition, experienced nursing staff can be empowered to make autonomous decisions.

Box 4.1 **A checklist of patients in whom sedation can often be safely reduced by nurses or trainee doctors without senior medical review**

- Patient requiring FiO_2 <0.5
- Patient established on a spontaneously triggered ventilation mode (e.g. pressure support ventilation; assisted spontaneous breathing)
- Positive end-expiratory pressure <10 cmH$_2$O
- No (or minor) requirement for cardiovascular support with vasopressors or inotropic drugs
- No evidence of ongoing haemorrhage or hypovolaemia
- Not experiencing uncontrolled hypertension, myocardial ischaemia or arrhythmias
- No problems with intracranial pressure
- No unstable fractures or cervical spine injury
- Cooperative non-agitated patient
- Adequate pain control

Sedation breaks

A sedation break is a period during which continuous sedation is stopped, usually until the patient regains consciousness. Once the patient is conscious the need for further sedation is re-evaluated, and it is only reintroduced if necessary. Sedation breaks are best linked to assessment of ventilatory function and potential for weaning. Several randomized trials have shown that a daily sedation break can decrease the duration of coma and mechanical ventilation, and

improve a range of patient outcomes. This approach is particularly valuable in avoiding accumulation of sedative drugs in patients with organ dysfunction. Sedation breaks are often included in protocols, for example on a daily basis.

Sedation monitors

These monitors are designed to measure conscious level. Most devices, such as the Bispectral Index (BIS), were developed for depth of anaesthesia monitoring rather than for use in the critically ill patient in intensive care. Although the output from these devices correlates with sedation state, they have poor discrimination for different sedation states and are not widely used. There is no evidence that these monitors are more effective than clinical protocols.

Withdrawing sedation

Some common problems encountered during sedation withdrawal are listed in Table 4.4. Delirium is described in more detail below. For most intensive care patients stopping sedation does not cause a physiological withdrawal syndrome, although this can occur in patients who have required large doses of sedative and analgesic drugs, especially for prolonged periods. Sedation withdrawal syndromes typically include tachycardia, hypertension, sweating and agitation. If this occurs, a more gradual withdrawal of the drugs is needed. Switching to a different drug class, especially α_2-agonists such as clonidine, may be an effective strategy to smooth out the features of withdrawal syndromes.

Delirium

Delirium is an acute fluctuating change in mental status characterized by sensory inattention and altered conscious level. Up to

Score	Term	Description	
+4	Combative	Overtly combative, violent, immediate danger to staff	
+3	Very agitated	Pulls or removes tube(s) or catheter(s); aggressive	
+2	Agitated	Frequent nonpurposeful movement, fights ventilator	
+1	Restless	Anxious but movements not aggressive or vigorous	
0	Alert and calm		
−1	Drowsy	Not fully alert, but has sustained awakening (eye opening/eye contact) to voice (>10 seconds)	Verbal stimulation
−2	Light sedation	Briefly awakens with eye contact to voice (<10 seconds)	
−3	Moderate sedation	Movement or eye opening to voice (but no eye contact)	
−4	Deep sedation	No response to voice, but movement or eye opening to physical stimulation	Physical stimulation
−5	Unarousable	No response to voice or physical stimulation	

Procedure for RASS assessment
1. Observe patient
   - Patient is alert, restless, or agitated. Score 0 to +4
2. If not alert, state patient's name and say to open eyes and look at speaker.
   - Patient awakens with sustained eye opening and eye contact. Score −1
   - Patient awakens with eye opening and eye contact, but not sustained. Score −2
   - Patient has any movement in response to voice but no eye contact. Score −3
3. When no response to verbal stimulation, physically stimulate patient by shaking shoulder and/or rubbing sternum.
   - Patient has any movement to physical stimulation. Score −4
   - Patient has no response to any stimulation. Score −5

Figure 4.1 The Richmond Agitation–Sedation Scale (RASS) for assessing clinical sedation status among critically ill patients. From Ely *et al.* JAMA 289 (2003). Copyright (2003) American Medical Association. All rights reserved.

Table 4.4 Common problems associated with sedation withdrawal.

Problem	Possible causes	Solution
Agitated patient	Pain Delirium Physiological withdrawal syndrome Inadequate oxygenation/ventilation	Ensure adequate analgesia Haloperidol; minimize precipitating factors Staged drug withdrawal; adjuvant drugs, e.g. α_2-agonists Review ventilator settings; ensure patient-ventilator synchronization; ensure adequate FiO_2 and mechanical support
Failure to regain consciousness	Accumulation of sedative drugs/active metabolites Encephalopathy (septic; metabolic; hepatic etc) Undiagnosed neuropathology (e.g. cerebrovascular event)	Sedation hold until conscious level improves Treat underlying condition; sedation hold; EEG if delayed recovery A thorough neurological examination should be performed, particularly looking for focal neurological signs with asymmetry of pupils or limb reflexes. Brain imaging (CT scan) is much more likely to reveal a structural lesion in the presence of these signs; treat appropriately

80% of ICU patients may suffer delirium, and this often becomes clinically apparent when sedative drugs are reduced or stopped. Of these, <10% have an agitated delirium, which is relatively easy to recognize. The majority have hypoactive delirium, which frequently passes unrecognized. Some risk factors for delirium are listed in Table 4.5. Delirium is associated with adverse outcomes from critical illness including adverse psychological outcomes, and with higher illness costs.

Diagnosing delirium

A common barrier to diagnosing delirium, especially hypoactive delirium, is the presence of mechanical ventilation and/or

Table 4.5 Some factors increasing the risk of delirium.

Drugs	Benzodiazepines; anticholinergics; antihistamines; steroids; metoclopramide
Infection	Sepsis syndrome; hospital acquired infections; central nervous system infections
Metabolic disturbances	Electrolyte disturbances; hypo/hyperglycaemia; renal failure; hepatic failure
Age	Older age (especially >70 years)
Drug withdrawal	Alcohol; opioids; sedative drugs; nicotine
Known neuropathology	Cerebrovascular disease; dementia
Sleep disturbance	Sleep deprivation
Environment	Lack of natural light; poor lighting; loss of day/night discrimination; excessive environmental noise

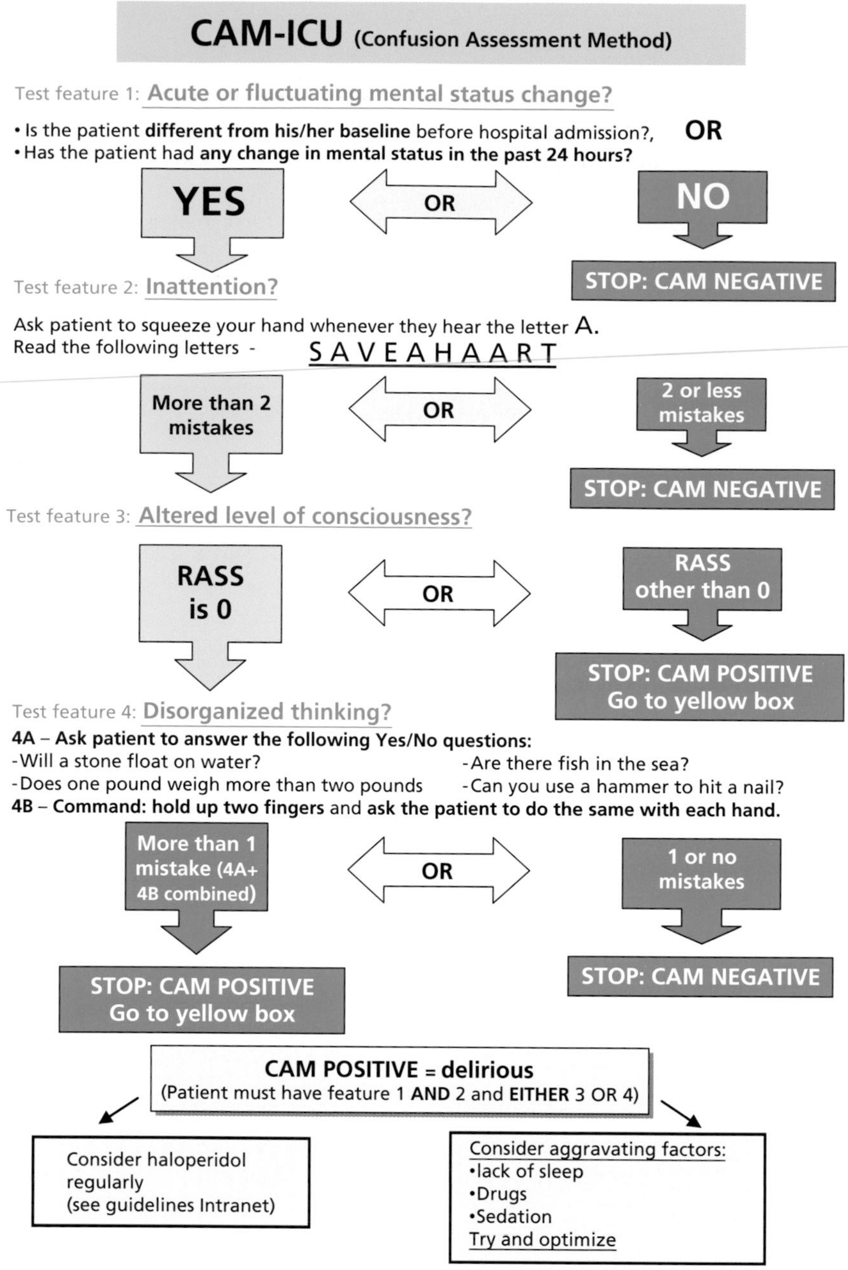

CAM-ICU (Confusion Assessment Method)

Test feature 1: Acute or fluctuating mental status change?

• Is the patient **different from his/her baseline** before hospital admission?, **OR**
• Has the patient had **any change in mental status in the past 24 hours?**

YES — OR — **NO**

NO → **STOP: CAM NEGATIVE**

Test feature 2: Inattention?

Ask patient to squeeze your hand whenever they hear the letter A.
Read the following letters - S A V E A H A A R T

More than 2 mistakes — OR — **2 or less mistakes**

2 or less mistakes → **STOP: CAM NEGATIVE**

Test feature 3: Altered level of consciousness?

RASS is 0 — OR — **RASS other than 0**

RASS other than 0 → **STOP: CAM POSITIVE Go to yellow box**

Test feature 4: Disorganized thinking?

4A – Ask patient to answer the following Yes/No questions:
- Will a stone float on water?
- Does one pound weigh more than two pounds
- Are there fish in the sea?
- Can you use a hammer to hit a nail?

4B – Command: hold up two fingers and ask the patient to do the same with each hand.

More than 1 mistake (4A+ 4B combined) — OR — **1 or no mistakes**

1 or no mistakes → **STOP: CAM NEGATIVE**

More than 1 mistake → **STOP: CAM POSITIVE Go to yellow box**

CAM POSITIVE = delirious
(Patient must have feature 1 **AND** 2 and **EITHER** 3 **OR** 4)

Consider haloperidol regularly
(see guidelines Intranet)

Consider aggravating factors:
• lack of sleep
• Drugs
• Sedation
Try and optimize

Figure 4.2 The Confusion Assessment Method for ICU (CAM-ICU) for recognition of delirium in the critically ill patient linked to Richmond Agitation–Sedation Scale sedation scoring.

sedative drugs, particularly during sedation withdrawal. This can make assessment of cognition difficult. The Confusion Assessment Method for ICU (CAM-ICU) is a validated tool that can identify delirium within 1–2 minutes, even in intubated patients. This can be linked and combined to the RASS score (Figures 4.1 and 4.2).

Managing delirium

Delirium can be logically managed using the flowchart shown in Figure 4.3. A key issue is to stop or avoid factors that perpetuate or exacerbate delirium, especially benzodiazepines; to correct reversible factors that could be contributory; and to switch to anti-psychotic agents (usually haloperidol) to manage agitation.

At present it is unclear whether patients with hypoactive delirium benefit from haloperidol treatment.

Sleep in intensive care

Sleep disturbance in the ICU is common. This results from many factors, some of which relate to the underlying illness (stress response, pain, inflammation, encephalopathy) and some from the environment (excessive noise, lighting, diagnostic and patient care activities). Normal sleep is typically disrupted resulting in increased sleep fragmentation, an increase in Stages 1 and 2 sleep, and decreases in Stages 3 and 4 sleep and REM sleep. Overall, sleep deprivation is common and circadian sleep rhythms disturbed.

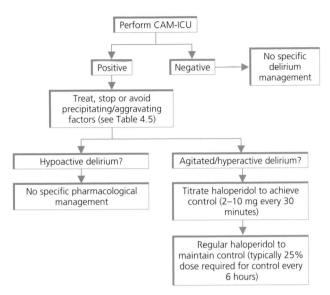

Figure 4.3 A stepwise approach to assessing and managing the delirious patient in the intensive care unit.

Optimizing sleep involves minimizing contributory environmental factors such as noise and physical disturbances. Optimizing patient–ventilator synchronization also decreases sleep disturbance. The role of sedatives is controversial. Benzodiazepines and other sedative drugs may prolong or increase sleep disturbance, and night-time 'sleep' should not be induced with sedative infusions. Newer non-benzodiazepine agents, such as zopiclone, may disrupt normal sleep patterns to a lesser degree. The role of melatonin is currently unclear.

Summary

Provision of sedation is one of the commonest ICU interventions. There is strong evidence that a systematic method for assessing and managing sedation using clinical tools and protocols can improve patient outcomes and quality of care. Distinguishing the need for sedative drugs from the presence of delirium is increasingly recognized as important for avoiding unnecessarily prolonged sedation in the ICU.

Further reading

Ely EW, Inouye SK, Bernard GR, *et al.* Delirium in mechanically ventilated patients: validity and reliability of the confusion assessment method for the intensive care unit (CAM-ICU). *JAMA* 2001; 286:2703–10

Ely EW, Truman B, Shintani A, Gordon S, *et al.* Monitoring sedation status over time in ICU patients – Reliability and validity of the Richmond Agitation-Sedation Scale (RASS). *JAMA* 2003; 289:2983–91.

Friese RS. Sleep and recovery from critical illness and injury: A review of theory, current practice, and future directions. *Crit Care Med* 2008; 36:697–705.

Girard TD, Kress JP, Fuchs BD, *et al.* Efficacy and safety of a paired sedation and ventilator weaning protocol for mechanically ventilated patients in intensive care (Awakening and Breathing Controlled trial): a randomised controlled trial. *Lancet* 1008; 371:126–34.

Sessler CN, Varney K. Patient-focussed sedation and analgesia in the ICU. *Chest* 2008; 133:522–65.

Online tutorial

There is an online tutorial on this subject at http://www.scottish intensive-care.org.uk/education/index.htm. Click on the 'Induction tutorials' tab to find it.

CHAPTER 5

Pathophysiology of Organ Failure

Charles Hinds[1] *and Mervyn Singer*[2]

[1] Barts and The London Queen Mary School of Medicine, London, UK
[2] University College London, London, UK

OVERVIEW

- Single organ failure may arise as a result of a direct insult (e.g. pulmonary aspiration). Failure of one organ may impinge secondarily on others (e.g. renal and respiratory failure following cardiogenic shock). Multiple organ failure can follow an uncontrolled systemic inflammatory response to a triggering insult (e.g. trauma, infection)

- Multiple organ failure is precipitated by dissemination of a dysregulated pro- and anti-inflammatory response to pathogen-associated or damage-associated molecular patterns (PAMPs and DAMPs)

- Downstream pathways involved in the development of organ failure include neural, endocrine, bioenergetic and metabolic

- Risk factors for the development of multiple organ failure include comorbidities (e.g. diabetes, cirrhosis, HIV infection, malnutrition, cancer, immunosuppressant therapy), smoking and alcohol excess, and genetic predisposition

- The mortality in patients who develop shock and multiple organ failure is high (60–70%)

- The importance of avoiding iatrogenic exacerbation of organ injury is increasingly recognized

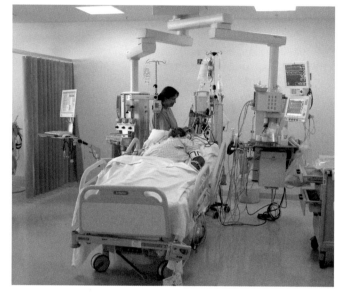

Figure 5.1 A patient with multiple organ failure.

Introduction

Patients are admitted to intensive care for any of a multitude of reasons. Some need intensive monitoring, specialized nursing and accurate titration of therapy with the aim of preventing deterioration and organ dysfunction. Others require intensive care for conditions specifically affecting a single organ, for example subarachnoid haemorrhage. Some have conditions affecting one organ that may then impinge secondarily on others, for example renal and respiratory failure following cardiogenic shock. Others are admitted with multiple organ failure following an uncontrolled systemic inflammatory response to a triggering insult (Figures 5.1 and 5.2)

Most commonly, the initiating event is infectious or traumatic (including surgery) (Box 5.1). Inflammation is an appropriate, and normally protective, host response designed to contain and resolve local tissue damage and repel microbial invasion. In some patients, however, this innate immune response is excessive, leading to systemic activation of pathways affecting multiple systems, for example hormonal, metabolic, bioenergetic, coagulation, that can progress to dysfunction or overt failure of one or more organs.

Box 5.1 **Examples of triggers of systemic inflammation**

- Infection
- Trauma (including surgery)
- Haemorrhage
- Burns
- Pancreatitis
- Drug or transfusion reaction
- Cardiac arrest
- Inhalation injury
- Hyperthermia and hypothermia
- Electrocution
- Near-drowning
- Poisons, toxins, insect bites

ABC of Intensive Care, Second Edition.
Edited by Graham R. Nimmo and Mervyn Singer.

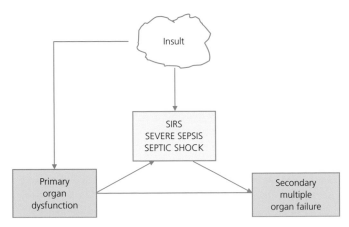

Figure 5.2 Progression from insult to organ failure.

A continuum exists from systemic inflammation (the systemic inflammatory response syndrome, SIRS) through to multiple organ dysfunction and shock. Box 5.2 provides definitions for these syndromes.

Box 5.2 **Definitions**

Systemic inflammatory response syndrome (SIRS)

Two or more of:

- Temperature $>38°C$ or $<36°C$
- Heart rate >90 bpm
- Respiratory rate >20 breaths/min or $PaCO_2$ <32 mmHg (4.3 kPa)
- WBC $>12\,000$ cells/mm^3, <4000 per mm^3 or $>10\%$ immature forms

Sepsis

- The systemic response to infection. Definition as for SIRS but as a result of infection.

Severe sepsis

Sepsis associated with organ dysfunction or hypoperfusion. Signs may include, but are not limited to, lactic acidosis, oliguria or an acute alteration in mental status.

Septic shock

Sepsis with hypotension, despite adequate fluid resuscitation and perfusion abnormalities.

Organ dysfunction

The presence of altered organ function in an acutely ill patient such that homeostasis cannot be maintained without intervention (transient impairment of organ function rapidly responsive to short-term measures should probably be excluded from this definition).

This standard terminology is an artificial construct. Nevertheless, it usefully illustrates how an inflammatory insult of whatever aetiology pursues a common path that can progress through the various stages of severity to culminate in similar histopathological, physiological and biochemical changes. It also highlights the increased mortality risk as the severity worsens, ranging from less than 10% for SIRS through to 30–50% for multiple organ failure, and 60–70%

if shock is also present. Sequential multiple organ failure is now the commonest modality of death in intensive care patients.

Different organs can be affected by this systemic inflammatory process and with varying degrees of severity. Sequential failure of vital organs occurs progressively over days to weeks. Single organ failure may predominate but, more commonly, organs are affected in combination. It is still unclear why the pattern varies between individuals and within the same patient over time. The term multiple organ dysfunction syndrome (MODS) has been suggested to indicate the wide range of severity and dynamic nature of this condition (Box 5.3).

Box 5.3 **Characteristic clinical features of patients with MODS**

- An increased metabolic rate (early stages)
- A hyperdynamic circulation (though may be markedly depressed)
- Hyperventilation
- An impaired immune response
- Hypotension

Organ failures in MODS

Lung (often first organ to be affected)
- ALI/ARDS
- Ventilator associated pneumonia (further stimulus to inflammation)

Cardiovascular
- Initial hyperdynamic circulation
- Vasodilatation, myocardial depression, hypotension, eventual cardiovascular collapse with failure to deliver/utilize oxygen at the tissue level

Kidney (commonly affected)
- Acute kidney injury

Liver (frank hepatic failure unusual)
- Jaundice, elevated liver enzymes, hypoalbuminaemia

Gastrointestinal (common)
- Inability to tolerate enteral feeds, large gastric aspirates, paralytic ileus, abdominal distension, diarrhoea
- Haemorrhage, ischaemic colitis, acalculous cholecystitis, pancreatitis

Central nervous system
- Impaired conscious level, delirium, coma, "septic encephalopathy"

Peripheral nervous system
- Critical illness polyneuromyopathy

Haematological
- Coagulopathy
- Disseminated intravascular coagulation
- Bone marrow failure

Metabolic/endocrine
- Elevated blood sugar levels, catabolism, wasting

There is now a considerable body of evidence to suggest that susceptibility to infectious diseases and sepsis, and outcome from these conditions, is influenced by inherited DNA sequence variations.

Single nucleotide polymorphisms in promoter or coding regions of genes that mediate or control innate immunity and the inflammatory response have been primarily implicated. Precise and convincing identification of the explanatory genes and polymorphisms has, however, proved to be elusive. Much larger studies than those performed to date, with more comprehensive (genome-wide) genotyping, replication of positive findings and allied functional studies will be required to resolve these uncertainties. The role of other structural variants (e.g. copy number variation, rare variants) and epigenetic changes will also require investigation.

Other risk factors for SIRS, sepsis and MODS include comorbidities such as diabetes, cirrhosis, HIV infection, malnutrition, cancer, medications (e.g. immunosuppressants) and alcohol in excess, all of which may compromise immunity. Diminished cardiovascular reserve can exacerbate tissue hypoperfusion and amplify the inflammatory response. The immune response also varies markedly with age, making the patient either more or less prone to specific infections.

Precise mechanisms underlying the pathophysiology of multi-organ injury remain to be fully elucidated (Figure 5.3). It is known that specific molecular signatures from pathogens (PAMPs) and tissue injury (DAMPs) are recognized by extra- and intracellular receptors sited on or within macrophages, circulating immune cells and endothelial cells. The best known is the Toll-like receptor family, of which 10 have been characterized in man.

These detect bacteria, fungi, viruses and parasites, and damaged cell constituents that have escaped their normal milieu (e.g. mitochondrial fragments). Through a series of phosphorylation cascades they stimulate production of many transcription factors of which the most studied is nuclear factor kappa-B (Figure 5.4).

These transcription factors enter the nucleus and affect the expression of genes encoding proteins responsible for initiating, propagating and also quenching the inflammatory response. Whereas many gene transcripts show increased expression, the majority are downregulated. There are also many post-transcriptional changes that affect the production of proteins, and the activities and concentration of enzymes.

In those who develop organ failure, many inflammatory mediators are produced in excess. These include cytokines (e.g. tumour necrosis factor, and interleukins-1 and -6) and other molecules (e.g. nitric oxide). Cell surface receptors may be up- or downregulated. There may be local effects from these mediators or release/overspill into the blood and lymphatics affecting distant organs and stimulating immune cells. As an example, neutrophils are activated to migrate across the blood vessel wall into tissue spaces where they degranulate, releasing reactive oxygen species and proteases. Whereas in a normal situation these are important mechanisms for attacking microbes, here they may damage healthy host tissue. Some mediators (e.g. bradykinin, prostanoids) also increase vascular leak, aiding not only the passage of immune cells out of the circulation,

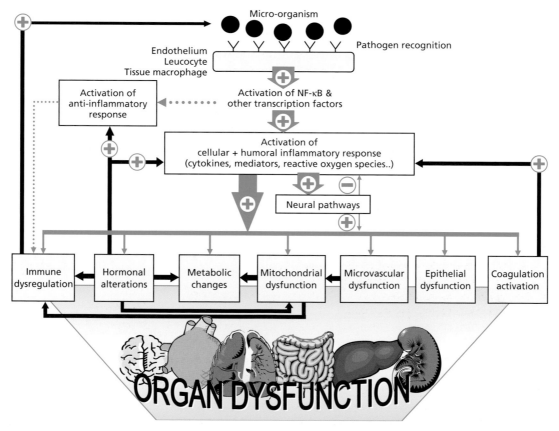

Figure 5.3 Systems pathways contributing to organ dysfunction in sepsis. *Source:* From Abraham, E & Singer, M (2007). Mechanisms of sepsis-induced organ dysfunction. *Critical Care Medicine*, 35(10):2408–16. Reproduced with permission from Wolters Kluwer Health.

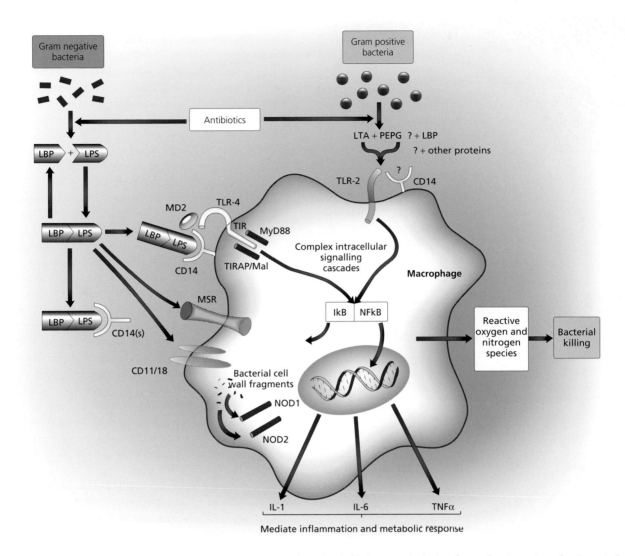

Figure 5.4 Induction of cytokine synthesis by the lipopolysaccharide–lipopolysaccharide-binding protein (LPS-LBP) complex. From *Intensive Care: A Concise Textbook*, 3rd edn, Hinds, C.J. and Watson, D. (eds). (2008) Saunders Elsevier.

but also encouraging the formation of interstitial oedema. In an attempt at healing, some organs mount a fibrotic response that can be severe and even permanent. Inflammatory cell infiltrate, interstitial oedema, local damage and fibrosis are the hallmarks of inflammation. Apart from vascular leak, blood vessels are generally dilated and their ability to constrict in response to catecholamines also diminishes. The net consequence is a hypovolaemic, vasodilated and hyporeactive circulation that, in an advanced state, is associated with severe hypotension. In concert with organ hypoperfusion and/or dysfunction, this is termed 'vasodilatory shock'.

These pathological features are seen in many organs including gut, liver and lung. In the lung, the most severe form (based on the severity of hypoxaemia) is termed the 'acute respiratory distress syndrome' (ARDS), whereas the milder manifestation is designated 'acute lung injury' (ALI) (Figure 5.5).

Mention should also be made of the commonplace feature of coagulopathy. In its most severe form, this can manifest as disseminated intravascular coagulation (DIC). However, despite its name, widespread micro- or macrocirculatory clots are relatively rare. The contribution of DIC to organ failure probably arises from the generation of thrombin, which is a potent pro-inflammatory stimulant, and from further endothelial activation.

The body attempts to quench the flames of inflammation by mounting an anti-inflammatory response with production of anti-inflammatory cytokines, mediators and downregulation of receptors (Figure 5.6). This actually commences early in the inflammatory process but may eventually predominate, pushing the patient into a state of endogenous immunosuppression. With the lines, tubes, drains and catheters of modern intensive care penetrating skin and other barriers, and the not-infrequent use of immunomodulatory therapy (including steroids, sedatives, catecholamines and gastric protectants) the patient is now at greatly increased risk of secondary infection and further bouts of inflammation.

The story becomes yet more complex. Often the extent of local inflammation, tissue damage and cell death, be it apoptotic or

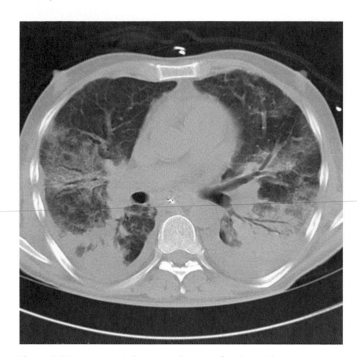

Figure 5.5 Lung computed tomography scan of patient with acute respiratory distress syndrome showing ground-glass opacification in non-dependent regions with atelectasis and consolidation in dependent regions. There are small pleural effusions.

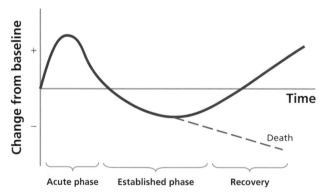

Figure 5.6 Fluctuation in pathway activation during the inflammatory process.

necrotic, is insufficient to account for the degree of physiological and biochemical organ dysfunction. In many instances, organs that have clearly failed on clinical grounds look remarkably normal histologically. For example, the term 'acute tubular necrosis' has conventionally been used to describe acute renal failure but this histological appearance is rarely, if ever, seen. A further conundrum is the ability of 'failed' organs to recover, often within days to weeks, and even when their regenerative capability is known to be poor, such as is the case for the kidney.

Clearly, an alternative yet complementary paradigm must be sought to reconcile these observations. It is therefore worth considering the potential role of pathways other than those involved in the inflammatory and immune cascades in the development of multi-organ dysfunction.

Neural regulation is increasingly recognized as playing a key role in controlling the body's response to stress, as well as in the development of organ failure. Activation of sympathetic and parasympathetic pathways and the hypothalamic–pituitary–adrenal axis are crucial aspects of the body's defence mechanisms. However, over-activation can have deleterious effects on organ function. Work stretching back 70–80 years clearly demonstrates a fundamental role of the neuroendocrine system in generating widespread end-organ damage from a variety of stressors, be they physical (e.g. infection, trauma, strenuous exercise, temperature disturbances) or even psychological (e.g. severe emotional stress).

Neural activation triggers a hormonal response that is, at least initially, in keeping with the needs of the body to defend itself against an external insult. There is increased production of catabolic hormones, such as adrenaline and cortisol, that increase tissue blood flow, mobilize substrates and modulate inflammation. Anabolic hormones are less important to sustain life acutely so their production falls or is directly antagonized. An example is insulin resistance with subsequent hyperglycaemia. Although beneficial in the sense that glucose is more freely available as a substrate for vital organs, the high blood sugar levels may themselves be damaging through glycation of proteins, increased generation of reactive oxygen species, immune suppression and enhanced bacterial growth.

Similarly, release of endogenous catecholamines can have deleterious consequences. Although necessary to sustain and distribute blood flow to vital organs and maintain an adequate blood pressure, they can also impair the immune response, cause direct tissue damage (notably to the heart), stimulate intravascular thrombosis and decrease metabolic efficiency.

Later, there is often a decrease in hormone production and/or receptor responsiveness. Notable examples include inappropriately low vasopressin levels, diminished thyroid hormone production (the 'low T3 syndrome'), vascular hyporeactivity to catecholamines and relative adrenal insufficiency. Many other hormones are affected, for example sex hormones, as well as gut hormones and adipokines that determine appetite (e.g. leptin). While these hormones may appear unconnected to acute inflammation, they play a crucial role in modulating and regulating the body's immune, bioenergetic and metabolic responses.

Metabolism also fluctuates in line with the phasic response to inflammation. Early in the inflammatory process, total body oxygen consumption increases. However, with increasing disease severity, this declines towards normal 'healthy' levels. Only in the recovery phase does a rebound rise in metabolism occur to support the healing process. An analogy could be made to hibernation (cold climates) or estivation (hot, arid environments), when the animal goes into a state of metabolic shutdown to optimize its chances of survival. Whether this metabolic shutdown is a direct effect or secondary to reduced energy provision related to mitochondrial dysfunction remains to be determined.

A further consequence of deranged metabolism is a decreased ability to utilize exogenous nutrients. This, combined with poor appetite and the frequent occurrence of gut dysfunction requires the body to mobilize endogenous stores, in particular fat and muscle. The loss of lean body mass, in part due to the inflammatory process that can lead to a critical illness myopathy, in part to prolonged immobilization and in part to auto-cannibalization, can result in severe muscle wasting, weakness and debility. This may compromise the surviving patient's ability to make a smooth recovery, including weaning from the ventilator and subsequent mobilization. A concurrent neuropathy (motor and/or sensory) may further compound this problem. Indeed, critical illness polymyoneuromyopathy may render the patient almost totally immobile for weeks, and weakness can persist for months or years.

In addition, we are belatedly recognizing that our efforts to maintain what we consider to be an appropriate level of homeostasis may actually compromise the body's attempts to cope with severe, prolonged inflammation or may even contribute to it. Large tidal volumes, high caloric input, blood transfusion and aggressive attempts to achieve 'normal' or 'supra-normal' values of cardiac output and oxygen delivery are but four examples of clear harm we have inflicted upon the critically ill patient. We now strive to avoid iatrogenic organ injury by aiming to achieve that which is achievable for that patient: 'acceptably abnormal' values.

In summary, we have highlighted the complexity of the fluctuating processes that culminate in organ failure. Early intervention to prevent organ failures and the avoidance of harm are the keys to success. Treating the cause is pivotal. Hopefully, a better understanding of the underlying pathophysiology will further improve outcomes, although definitive answers are some way off.

Further reading

Abraham EA, Singer M. Mechanisms of sepsis-induced organ dysfunction. *Crit Care Med* 2007; 35:2408–16.

Annane D, Bellissant E, Cavaillon J-M. Septic shock. *Lancet* 2005; 365: 63–78.

Hotchkiss RS, Karl IE. The pathophysiology and treatment of sepsis. *N Engl J Med* 2003; 348:138–50.

Medzhitov R. Inflammation 2010: new adventures of an old flame. *Cell* 2010; 140:771–6.

CHAPTER 6

Severe Sepsis

Michael Gillies[1] *and Duncan Wyncoll*[2]

[1] Royal Infirmary of Edinburgh, Edinburgh, UK
[2] Guy's and St Thomas' Hospital, London, UK

> **OVERVIEW**
> - In the developed world, more people die from severe sepsis per year than heart disease or stroke
> - Severe sepsis results from an excessive innate response to an external infectious stimulus
> - Clinical features of severe sepsis are varied and often relate to the precipitating infective cause
> - Correction of hypoxaemia with early fluid resuscitation and immediate antibiotics with effective source control form the cornerstone of the initial management of sepsis
> - Delayed or inadequate initial management adversely affects outcome
> - Patients with severe sepsis should be managed in a critical care setting

Introduction

Sepsis results from the interaction between the host response and the presence of micro-organisms and/or their toxins within the body. Simplistically, it is often thought of as a spillover of an initially local inflammatory process into the systemic circulation. An infective source is formally identified in approximately 65% of patients with sepsis, but blood cultures are only positive in 25%. Severe sepsis (i.e. sepsis with concurrent organ dysfunction) can be rapidly progressive and, if not treated promptly, results in multiple organ failure and death.

The incidence of severe sepsis has increased steadily over recent years. In some countries up to 50% of intensive care unit (ICU) patients have sepsis at the time of admission or develop it during their stay. The worldwide incidence is thought to be about 1.8 million cases annually, with the European Union incidence estimated to be approximately 90 cases per 100 000. Poor recognition of the syndrome and the absence of a clear definition and a simple diagnostic test, means that this figure may be an underestimate. In the developed world severe sepsis is associated with more deaths per year than heart disease or stroke.

ABC of Intensive Care, Second Edition.
Edited by Graham R. Nimmo and Mervyn Singer.
© 2011 Blackwell Publishing Ltd. Published 2011 by Blackwell Publishing Ltd.

Definition

In 1991 the American College of Chest Physicians and the US Society of Critical Care Medicine produced a consensus document defining sepsis and the systemic inflammatory response syndrome (SIRS) (Table 6.1). Although these definitions have some major limitations, they are still widely used, particularly in clinical trials. Most importantly, this definition does not adequately stratify the very heterogeneous group that sepsis patients represent, and does not take account of the interaction between the infectious stimulus and the host response. In an attempt to address this, the PIRO system was proposed by a further consensus conference held in 2001 (Table 6.2).

The aetiology of SIRS can be related to an infectious or non-infectious cause (Figure 6.1). When SIRS is secondary to a documented or suspected infection it is known as 'sepsis', and when sepsis is associated with organ dysfunction, it is termed 'severe sepsis'. The term 'septic shock' implies persistent sepsis-induced hypotension (with associated tissue hypoxia) despite adequate fluid resuscitation.

Severe sepsis is predominantly caused by bacteria, but fungi and viruses are also occasionally implicated. The most common sources of severe sepsis include:

- pneumonia (community or hospital acquired)
- intra-abdominal infection, for example appendicitis, bowel perforation and peritonitis, bowel infarction, abscess or cholangitis
- urinary tract infection, for example pyelonephritis
- skin and soft tissue infection
- catheter-related blood stream infection, for example vascular access device
- central nervous system infection, for example meningitis (Figure 6.2)
- endocarditis.

Many cases of severe sepsis are community acquired, but the incidence of hospital-acquired infection is steadily increasing. Hospital-acquired infections are more frequently associated with resistant organisms, and a good knowledge of local antimicrobial resistance patterns is vital in order to select the most appropriate treatment from the outset.

Gram-positive cocci and Gram-negative bacilli are the microbes most commonly implicated in the pathogenesis of sepsis, with components of the bacterial cell wall triggering the inflammatory

Table 6.1 American College of Chest Physicians/Society of Critical Care Medicine consensus definition of systemic inflammatory response syndrome (SIRS) and sepsis.

SIRS	Two or more of: Temperature $<36°C$ *or* $>38°C$ Heart rate >90 bpm Respiratory rate >20 *or* $PaCO_2 > 4.5$ kPa *or* mechanically ventilated White cell count $<4× 10^9$ *or* $>12× 10^9$ *or* $>10\%$ immature forms
Sepsis	SIRS plus documented *or* suspected infection
Severe sepsis	Sepsis plus organ dysfunction *or* hypoperfusion (e.g. hyperlactataemia, oliguria or hypotension)
Septic shock	Sepsis with hypotension (systolic blood pressure <90 mmHg or need for vasopressor infusion) despite adequate fluid resuscitation

Table 6.2 The PIRO classification.

Predisposition	Past medical history Genetic predisposition Age
Insult or infection	Known pathogens Amenable to surgery/source control Non-infectious precipitants Gene profile
Response	SIRS/sepsis Shock and hypoperfusion Markers: Impaired host response (e.g. HLA-DR) Activated inflammatory process (e.g. CRP, PCT) Therapy targets (e.g. protein C)
Organ dysfunction	Number of organ systems failing

CRP, C-reactive protein; PCT, procalcitonin.

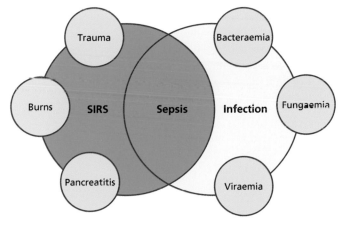

Figure 6.1 Causes of systemic inflammatory response syndrome and sepsis.

processes. However, viruses, fungi and atypical bacteria can trigger an identical response.

As described in more detail in Chapter 5, microbial components bind to specialized receptors on immune and endothelial cells. Activation of these receptors in turn trigger transcription factors such as nuclear factor kappa B (NFkB), resulting in secretion of

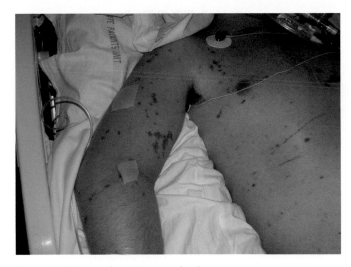

Figure 6.2 Patient with meningococcal rash.

a variety of pro- and anti-inflammatory mediators and receptors. Examples include cytokines, such as interleukins 1, 2 and 6 (IL-1, IL-2, IL-6) and tumour necrosis factor alpha (TNF-α), arachidonic acid metabolites, such as prostaglandins and thromboxanes, and endogenous gases, such as nitric oxide and carbon monoxide. These mediators activate leucocytes and the endothelium, activate the coagulation network, and trigger a variety of metabolic and hormonal effects. Activation and amplification of these multiple cascades lead to the clinical features of the sepsis syndrome.

Vasodilation induced by NO and other molecules leads to hypotension and impaired perfusion whereas disruption of the endothelium leads to generalized oedema and hypovolaemia. Derangements in macro- and microcirculatory flow therefore result in failure of adequate oxygen delivery to the tissues and the consequent tissue hypoxia further amplifies the inflammatory response. Similarly, although intravascular clots are rarely seen, there is significant thrombin generation, another potent pro-inflammatory stimulus. It is also likely that in established sepsis tissue oxygen utilization is impaired at the mitochondrial level. Untreated, this cycle of inflammation, poor perfusion, coagulopathy and impaired oxygen utilization leads to multiple organ dysfunction and, potentially, death.

Clinical presentation and diagnosis

The clinical features of sepsis are varied and often relate to the precipitating cause. In classic sepsis the patient is warm, flushed and vasodilated with signs of SIRS. However, the presentation can be insidious and non-specific, especially in elderly people or those with multiple comorbidities, when it may present with cold peripheries and a hypodynamic cardiovascular response. In this situation, severe sepsis may be misdiagnosed as, for example, cardiogenic shock or pulmonary embolism.

Most typically the following features are present.

Cardiovascular failure

Patients with sepsis are usually warm, flushed and vasodilated. They are frequently hyperdynamic, tachycardic and hypotensive with a high cardiac output, although this may require prior fluid resuscitation. Signs suggestive of reduced tissue perfusion and oxygen supply, that is elevated serum lactate and low central venous oxygen saturation (ScvO$_2$) may also be present. The rise in lactate seen in sepsis partly reflects increased catecholamine-driven aerobic glycolysis in addition to the traditional recognized tissue hypoxia and anaerobic metabolism. Two phases of septic shock are described 'warm shock' (as described above) and so-called 'cold shock' characterized by signs of poor peripheral perfusion and low cardiac output. Patients with cold shock have an inadequate cardiac output and typically require further fluid resuscitation and inotropic support to correct hypovolaemia and/or sepsis-induced myocardial depression.

Respiratory failure

Tachypnoea and increased minute ventilation are early signs of severe sepsis and may indicate the onset of respiratory failure. This relates to increasing metabolic acidosis and the development of non-cardiogenic pulmonary oedema from increased capillary leak, which may result in progressive hypoxaemia and respiratory failure. Acute lung injury occurs frequently in this group, and many patients require ventilatory support as fatigue ensues.

Renal dysfunction

Acute kidney injury may accompany sepsis. It is in part related to concurrent hypotension and hypovolaemia, but also directly to the inflammatory process. Oliguria is an early sign and adequate fluid resuscitation does not always reverse this. In about 5–10% of cases of severe sepsis, oliguria progresses to anuric renal failure and renal replacement therapy (RRT) is required. This is usually provided as continuous haemo(dia)filtration or daily intermittent haemodialysis. When the episode of sepsis has resolved renal function recovers in well over 90% of patients with normal renal function before the septic insult.

Sepsis-associated encephalopathy/neuropathy

Cerebral dysfunction can manifest as confusion, agitation or coma. It is an early sign, often present at the onset of other signs of organ failure. In addition, the patient may develop autonomic dysfunction, peripheral neuropathy (motor and/or sensory) and/or myopathy – 'critical illness polyneuropathy/myopathy'. These complications may be particularly severe and may sometimes fail to recover, even in long-term survivors.

Haematological failure

Prolongation of the prothrombin and activated partial thromboplastin time, thrombocytopenia and deficiencies of protein C, antithrombin or tissue factor pathway inhibitor may also be present in severe sepsis patients. In the most extreme form, disseminated intravascular coagulation may develop, but this is now a relatively unusual clinical manifestation.

Gastrointestinal dysfunction

Ileus, bowel dysfunction and, potentially, bacterial translocation from the gut to the systemic circulation may occur as a result of sepsis. Biochemical evidence of liver dysfunction is often seen, and impaired liver function results in reduced lactate clearance and altered drug handling.

Biomarkers

Among many others, C-reactive protein, procalcitonin, protein C and IL-6 levels have all been proposed as biomarkers for sepsis, either for diagnosis or early prognostication. At present, their usefulness is uncertain and their precise role in the management of patients is yet to be clearly defined.

Patient management

It is convenient to divide sepsis management into the initial resuscitation phase and the management phase. In 2008, the Surviving Sepsis Campaign (SSC) published updated guidelines. The campaign sought to both raise the profile of severe sepsis worldwide, and to standardize its treatment with a 6-hour 'resuscitation bundle' and a 24-hour 'management bundle'. An outline of these bundles is shown in Figure 6.3.

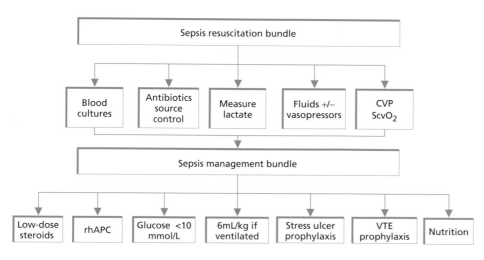

Figure 6.3 Surviving Sepsis Campaign 6- and 24-hour bundles.

	Assessment	Action	Investigations
A	Airway and conscious level – Maintaining own airway? Requiring intervention?	i. Open and clear ii. Chin life, head tilt iii. Airway adjunct iv. Advanced airway – CALL for HELP	Arterial blood gas (ABG)
B	Breathing – Look, listen and feel, rate, volume and symmetry, work of breathing and pattern	i. High concentration O_2 (60–100%) ii. Monitor SpO_2 iii. Ventilate if required ➤ O_2 concentration is determined by type of mask as well as flow from wall/cylinder and patients respiratory rate*	Chest X-ray (CXR)
C	Circulation – Pulse rate/volume, rhythm/character Skin colour and temp Capillary refill Blood pressure	i. Monitor ECG and BP ii. IV access iii. Fluid bolus iv. Vasoactive drugs – CALL for HELP	ECG
D	CNS and Conscious level – AVPU, GCS, pupil reaction Focal neurological signs	i. ABC and consider cause ➤ Hypoxaemia should always be treated first.	Glucose blood cultures
E	Examine and assess evidence – temperature	i. Review TPR, drug and fluid charts ii. Interpret investigations and results	

Figure 6.4 Suggested framework for early management of sepsis.

Initial resuscitation (first 6 hours)

The initial approach to the septic patient (Figure 6.4) should include:

- assessment of a patient's airway and breathing
- administration of adequate supplemental oxygen
- securing of adequate vascular access to facilitate prompt fluid resuscitation
- early administration of appropriate antibiotics, with source control if indicated.

These interventions form the cornerstone of the initial management of sepsis and are time-critical with a direct bearing on patient outcome. It is recommended that antibiotics are administered within 3 hours of emergency department (ED) admission and within 1 hour of non-ED admission. Blood and other appropriate cultures should be sent prior to administration of antibiotics if possible, but there should not be unnecessary delay. The choice of antibiotics will depend on the nature of the infection and the local hospital policy. An anatomical site of infection or other diagnosis should be established within the first 6 hours if possible. If the infection is amenable to source control, for example drainage of an abscess or debridement of infected tissues, then the appropriate expert help should be sought.

Early goal-directed therapy is currently recommended for patients with severe sepsis, following a study conducted by Rivers *et al* in 2001. Early measurement of serum lactate and central venous oxygen saturation ($ScvO_2$) are key to initial management using this strategy. A low $ScvO_2$ (i.e. <65%) is suggestive of poor tissue perfusion. An elevated $ScvO_2$ (>75%) should be interpreted with caution in established sepsis since it may be indicate failure of oxygen utilisation rather than adequacy of tissue oxygen delivery.

Initial resuscitation should be with intravenous fluid: 20–40 mL/kg is often necessary. Transfusion of packed cells should be considered if the $ScvO_2$ remains low and the haematocrit is less than 30%. The SSC guidelines recommend aiming for a lactate of <4 mmol/L, a central venous pressure (CVP) of 8–12 mmHg and an $ScvO_2$ of >70%. Whatever endpoints are used, they should however be tailored to the individual patient, for example a young fit patient may not require a CVP of 8–12 mmHg and, conversely, a patient with heart failure may require higher CVP values. Insertion of an arterial line at an early stage can be invaluable. Not only does it allow close monitoring of mean arterial pressure, but also allows frequent atraumatic blood gas analysis.

If the mean arterial pressure (MAP) remains <65 mmHg despite adequate fluid resuscitation, vasopressors (e.g. noradrenaline) should be administered if there is ongoing evidence of poor perfusion. If a low cardiac output state is measured/suspected, an inotropic agent (e.g. dobutamine, adrenaline) should be considered. Evidence does not currently support the recommendation of one agent over another. The SSC guidelines also recommend consideration of a vasopressin infusion in patients with refractory shock.

Ongoing management

Patients with severe sepsis should be managed in a critical care setting. Appropriate thromboembolic and stress ulcer prophylaxis should be given. In patients who are mechanically ventilated, the tidal volumes should be limited to 6–8 mL/kg, and airway plateau pressures maintained ≤30 cmH_2O. Early enteral nutrition should be commenced, when possible.

There are several additional therapies that have been advocated in severe sepsis which may also improve outcome, yet these all remain controversial.

Recombinant human activated protein C

Recombinant human activated protein C (rh-APC) controls inflammation and improves microcirculatory flow in severe sepsis. The multicentre PROWESS study showed a reduction in mortality associated with rh-APC use. However, subsequent studies that examined lower risk and non-indicated populations confirmed that the drug should be reserved for adults with multiple organ dysfunction and at high risk of death. The major adverse effect of administration of rh-APC is bleeding so each patient should be risk assessed prior to administration and during use. An ongoing study known as PROWESS-Shock has the potential to resolve the continued controversy surrounding this therapy.

Corticosteroids

Corticosteroids have been used to treat severe sepsis and, in particular, septic shock for >30 years however controversy still surrounds their use. In the last 15 years the concept of relative adrenal insufficiency was postulated, that is a subgroup of septic shock patients with an inadequate adrenal response, diagnosed by an inadequate serum cortisol response to a corticotrophin stimulation test. The largest corticosteroid trial to date, CORTICUS, did not demonstrate a survival benefit, but did demonstrate more rapid shock reversal. The use of corticosteroids should be balanced against potential complications that include an increased incidence of secondary infection, hyperglycaemia and, possibly, an increased risk of critical illness polyneuro(myo)pathy.

Glucose control

Insulin also has anti-inflammatory properties and prevention of hyperglycaemia has been associated with a reduction in duration of ICU admission, acute renal failure and critical illness polyneuropathy. The optimum range for blood glucose is yet to be fully determined. Although single-centre studies from Leuven, Belgium, suggested that tight glucose control (4.5–6.1 mmol/L) was associated with the best outcomes, several large multicentre RCTs (e.g. NICE-SUGAR) have since challenged this view, especially as the risk of hypoglycaemia was significantly increased. The current consensus is to strenuously avoid both hypo- and hyperglycaemia and to target glucose levels of approximately 6–8 mmol/L.

Renal replacement therapy

Renal replacement therapy should be offered to patients with acute kidney injury if there is a good chance of patient recovery. There is currently no evidence favouring intermittent haemodialysis over continuous haemofiltration. The use of 'high-dose' haemofiltration had been hypothesized to remove pro-inflammatory mediators with potential benefit; however, there is currently insufficient evidence to recommend the use of this therapy.

Further Reading

Angus DC, Linde-Zwirble WT, Lidicker J, *et al*. Epidemiology of severe sepsis in the United States: analysis of incidence, outcome, and associated costs of care. *Crit Care Med* 2001; 29: 1303–10.

Dellinger RP, Levy MM, Carlet JM, *et al*. Surviving Sepsis Campaign: International guidelines for management of severe sepsis and septic shock: /??/2008. *Crit Care Med* 2008; 36: 296–327.

Finfer S, Chittock DR, Su SY, *et al*. Intensive versus conventional glucose control in critically ill patients. NICE-SUGAR Study Investigators. *N Engl J Med* 2009; 360: 1283–97.

Finfer S, Ranieri VM, Thompson BT, *et al*. Design, conduct, analysis and reporting of a multi-national placebo-controlled trial of activated protein C for persistent septic shock. *Intensive Care Med* 2008; 34: 1935–47.

Rivers E, Nguyen B, Havstad S, *et al*. Early goal-directed therapy in the treatment of severe sepsis and septic shock. *N Engl J Med* 2001; 345: 1368–77.

Online tutorial

There is an online tutorial on this subject at http://www.scottish intensive-care.org.uk/education/index.htm. Click on the 'Induction tutorials' tab to find it.

CHAPTER 7

Respiratory Support

Simon Baudouin[1] and Timothy W. Evans[2]

[1] Royal Victoria Infirmary, Newcastle, UK
[2] Royal Brompton Hospital, London, UK

OVERVIEW

- The majority of patients admitted to critical care units will require advanced respiratory support in the form of assisted ventilation

- Provision of appropriate oxygen therapy remains a priority in respiratory failure. A range of fixed and variable performance devices allows accurate titration to patient needs

- Continuous positive airway pressure is effective in improving oxygenation in some patients with diffuse lung problems, for example severe pulmonary oedema and *Pneumocystis* pneumonia

- Non-invasive ventilation improves outcome in mildly acidotic patients with exacerbations of chronic obstructive pulmonary disease

- Intubation in the unstable, critically ill patient can be very challenging and should only be performed by experienced and competent practitioners

- Ventilator-induced lung injury is caused by the use of high volume/pressure ventilation. 'Lung protective' ventilator strategies, with deliberate hypoventilation, are commonly used in the critically ill and improve outcome

- Most patients who require longer term ventilation will undergo tracheostomy

Introduction

Respiratory failure is defined as a reduced arterial oxygen tension (PaO_2), with or without elevated levels of carbon dioxide ($PaCO_2$). It represents one of the commonest problems necessitating intensive care unit (ICU) admission. Traditionally, respiratory failure has been classified according to rapidity of onset (acute and chronic) and by the presence of hypoxaemia ($PaO_2 < 8$ kPa, normal range 10–13.3 kPa) either with (type II) or without (type I) hypercapnia (normal range of $PaCO_2$ 4.8–6.1 kPa). In clinical practice, patients may progress from type I to type II respiratory failure as the underlying condition evolves and as the patient tires. Moreover, either type may complicate a wide variety of pathologies.

ABC of Intensive Care, Second Edition.
Edited by Graham R. Nimmo and Mervyn Singer.

Oxygen therapy

Oxygen is normally administered via fixed and variable performance devices (Table 7.1 and Figure 7.1). The categorization of the device is determined by the flow rate of gas supplied, the volume of the mask itself and the presence of holes or other entrainment systems. Fixed performance devices are designed to provide a constant and predictable inspired oxygen concentration, irrespective of the patient's ventilatory pattern. Variable performance devices provide an inspired oxygen concentration (FiO_2) that varies according to the gas flow rate and patient's ventilatory pattern. The peak inspiratory flow rate (PIFR) has a significant effect on the concentration of oxygen reaching the alveoli when variable performance devices are used. The more critically ill the patient and the faster the PIFR, the greater the dilution of inspired oxygen by entrained atmospheric air and therefore the lower the FiO_2.

Patients suffering from mild hypoventilation, diffusion hypoxaemia and mild ventilation/perfusion mismatch require only modest increases in FiO_2 (to 0.3 or 0.4), achieved by supplying a flow rate of 4 L/min to a variable performance device. However, in patients with chronic respiratory failure (predominantly but not exclusively caused by chronic obstructive pulmonary disease), ventilatory drive is stimulated by hypoxaemia. If this is relieved through

Table 7.1 Oxygen delivery systems.

Method of delivery	FiO₂ achieved	Type of patient
Nasal cannula (1–2 L/min)	0.24–0.30	Stable patients
Venturi mask	0.24–0.50	Type II respiratory failure and COPD
Partial rebreathing mask	0.60 to 0.80	Acute Type I respiratory failure, e.g. pneumonia, asthma and acute pulmonary oedema
Non-rebreathing reservoir mask	Up to 0.90	Severely hypoxaemic patients
Tight-fitting mask or helmet (e.g. CaStar hood) used for NIV	Up to 1.0	Severely hypoxaemic patients
Anaesthetic face mask or endotracheal tube	Up to 1.0	Patients requiring intubation

COPD, chronic obstructive pulmonary disease; NIV, non-invasive ventilation.

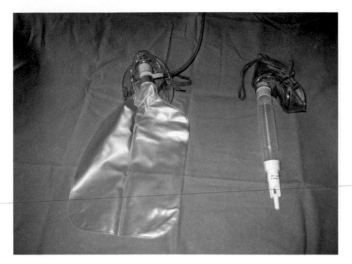

Figure 7.1 Two types of oxygen delivery devices. The reservoir device (on the left) enables the delivery of a high inspired oxygen concentration (FIO_2) (up to approximately 90%) whereas the Venturi device (on the right) delivers a fixed FIO_2.

the administration of oxygen at high FIO_2 via a variable performance device, arterial oxygen tension rises and respiratory drive is suppressed. The entrainment of room air is reduced, the proportion of oxygen inhaled increases, and respiratory drive is decreased further. The commonest reason for a rising $PaCO_2$ in the context of acute respiratory failure is respiratory muscle fatigue rather than loss of hypoxic respiratory drive: providing assisted ventilation is the appropriate response, not limiting oxygen provision.

An FIO_2 up to 0.85 can be achieved using oxygen flows of 10 L/min or greater, although considerable CO_2 rebreathing occurs if the oxygen supply falls or fails. Rebreathing can be eliminated and delivered FIO_2 increased still further if unidirectional valves are added to the circuitry. High oxygen concentrations inspired for prolonged periods may cause cellular toxicity and reabsorption atelectasis but may be necessary to maintain adequate levels of oxygenation.

Airway management

Ensuring the patient has a patent airway and adequate oxygen supply is a therapeutic priority in all circumstances. Head repositioning, removal of obstructions and insertion of a nasopharyngeal or oropharyngeal airway, and the application of positive pressure ventilation using an Ambu or other type of self-inflating bag–valve–mask apparatus may be needed to ensure airway patency and adequate ventilation. These manoeuvres can be applied equally effectively to the patient in respiratory distress as to the apnoeic patient. Ongoing respiratory support can be delivered to the conscious patient via a face mask to increase FIO_2, by applying continuous positive airway pressure (CPAP) or through intermittent positive pressure ventilation (IPPV) administered non-invasively (via nasal or full face mask). Patients with impaired conscious level require endotracheal intubation (Box 7.1 and Figures 7.2 and 7.3).

Box 7.1 Endotracheal intubation

The decision to intubate should be undertaken only by those possessing the relevant competencies in the use of anaesthetic, muscle relaxant and resuscitation drugs and advanced airway management. The decision to intubate is based on a number of factors including:

- Inability to maintain an airway (Glasgow Coma score of 8 or less)
- Exhaustion
- Deteriorating gas exchange, acid base status and respiratory rate
- Reversibility of underlying condition and premorbid condition

The equipment, anaesthetic and neuromuscular blocking agents required and the exact techniques employed are beyond the scope of this chapter.

Tracheostomy is appropriate in patients who require airway protection and secretion management, or prolonged periods of assisted ventilation. Sedation can be decreased, resistance to airflow is reduced and dead space diminished, aiding weaning from ventilatory support. Tracheostomy facilitates communication, feeding, and prevents the nasal, laryngeal and pharyngeal complications of intubation. The timing of insertion of tracheostomy remains controversial; an as yet unpublished UK multicentre trial showed no outcome difference between early (Day 4 of intubation or earlier) or late (on or after Day 10) insertion. The long-term risks of prolonged intubation such as subglottic stenosis, particularly in young females, have yet to be formally assessed.

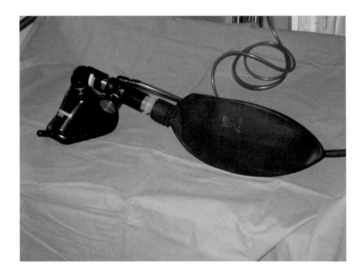

Figure 7.2 An anaesthetic type of full-face mask with a reservoir bag and unidirectional valve. This system will deliver an inspired oxygen concentration (FIO_2) of 100% and is suitable for manual ventilation of the critically ill before intubation.

Mechanical ventilatory support

Non invasive ventilatory support
Continuous positive airway pressure
CPAP generators produce a continuous positive pressure across the airway in spontaneously breathing patients (Figures 7.4 and 7.5). These devices require high oxygen/air flow rates to maintain a consistent pressure in the critically ill patient, and differ from

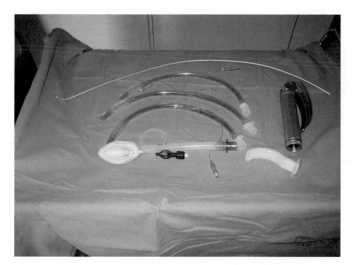

Figure 7.3 A selection of equipment required for intubation including a range of endotracheal tubes, a bougie for difficult intubations, a laryngoscope, an orophangeal airway and a laryngeal mask. Only competent and experienced practitioners should attempt to intubate the critically ill.

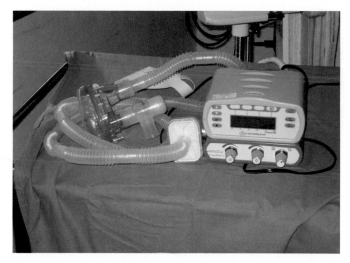

Figure 7.5 An alternative continuous positive airway pressure (CPAP) system that can be used on general wards. This requires a high-flow oxygen input and differs from the CPAP machines used to treat obstructive sleep apnoea.

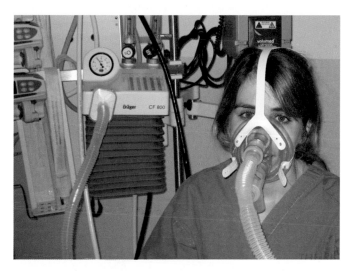

Figure 7.4 A full-face continuous positive airway pressure (CPAP) mask and CPAP machine. This device has a bellows to reduce flow variation during inspiration.

those used to treat ambulatory patients with obstructive sleep apnoea. A full facial mask provides a suitable interface, but requires careful fitting to ensure a good seal and avoid facial pressure sores and may render the patient claustrophobic. An alternative is the CPAP hood/helmet, which avoids the complication of pressure sores.

CPAP produces similar beneficial effects to positive-end respiratory pressure (PEEP) in the fully ventilated patient. It acts by 'recruiting' and then maintaining open collapsed and partially collapsed alveoli. Effective gas exchange is therefore restored with a reduction in shunt and an improvement in oxygenation. CPAP is most effective in diffuse lung disease with improvements in oxygen commonly occurring in severe pulmonary oedema and *Pneumocystis* pneumonia. In general, CPAP should not be used

in patients with significant airflow obstruction as it may lead to increased gas trapping. In addition, CPAP (like PEEP) may reduce venous return to the heart resulting in reduced cardiac output and hypotension. CPAP may increase the risk of pneumothoraces. The use of CPAP is not recommended in patients with a reduced conscious level in view of the risk of aspiration of gastric contents. In practice, it is well tolerated by most patients with few complications.

Non-invasive positive pressure ventilation

In the last 15 years, non-invasive positive pressure ventilation (NIV) has become established as an effective method of providing acute respiratory support to some groups of patients. The devices used to deliver NIV are true *ventilators* and should not be confused with

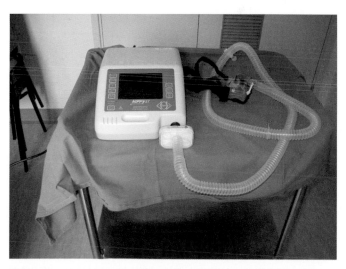

Figure 7.6 A non-invasive ventilator. These devices cycle from inspiration to expiration and have many of the features of the more complex critical care ventilators. They should be distinguished from continuous positive airway pressure machines, which cannot supply ventilatory support.

CPAP machines which do not cycle from inspiration to expiration (Figure 7.6). NIV devices tend to be smaller and more portable than standard intensive care ventilators. They have fewer features and lack some of the alarms of conventional machines, which may assist sleep. They usually use entrained oxygen rather than a dual air/oxygen mix. Most have a single inspiratory circuit, relying on either a hole or valve in the mask or tubing as the expiratory port (which *must* be present and not occluded). They can only deliver relatively low concentrations of oxygen and are not suitable for severely hypoxaemic patients.

NIV is a standard treatment in patients with acute exacerbations of COPD who develop an acute respiratory acidosis with a pH $\leqslant$ 7.35. Several randomized clinical trials have shown beneficial hospital outcomes attributed to the avoidance of intubation. In addition to patient preference there are a number of relative and absolute contraindications to NIV (Box 7.2). NIV may also be effective in other conditions causing acute respiratory failure, but its use should not delay intubation if required. In patients where the predicted clinical course of the disease process indicates that ventilatory support will be required for a prolonged period (e.g. 7–14 days) intubation of the trachea and ventilation via an endotracheal tube should not be delayed by the use of NIV, which may increase mortality. NIV (and CPAP) can be used successfully outside the critical care environment in selected cases, but training with support and escalation protocols must be in place to ensure patient safety.

Box 7.2 **Contraindications to NIV (adapted from the British Thoracic Society NIV guidelines)**

- facial burns/trauma/recent facial or upper airway surgery
- vomiting
- fixed upper airway obstruction
- undrained pneumothorax
- upper gastrointestinal surgery
- inability to protect the airway
- copious respiratory secretions
- life-threatening hypoxaemia
- haemodynamically unstable requiring inotropes/pressors (unless in a critical care unit)
- severe comorbidity
- confusion/agitation
- bowel obstruction

Invasive ventilatory support

IPPV is now applied via microprocessor-controlled mechanical ventilators (Figure 7.7). During inspiration the machine generates and delivers a flow of gas of pre-set FIO$_2$ into the lungs. This cycles to expiration after a given time period has elapsed (time cycling) or when a certain pressure is reached within the respiratory circuit (pressure cycling). The nature of the breath supplied can be modified by adjusting the flow rate with which the gas is delivered. The optimal mode of ventilation depends in part upon the nature of the underlying illness (particularly the presence or absence of pulmonary parenchymal or airway pathology), the phase of the

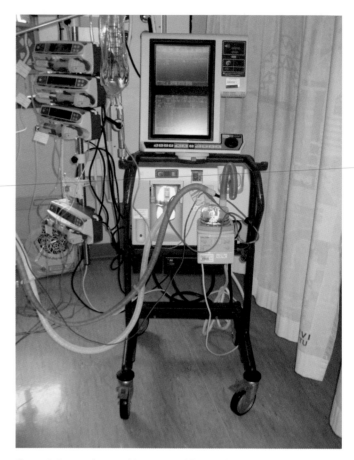

Figure 7.7 A modern, multiprogrammable critical care ventilator. These devices can delivery many different types of ventilation, including both pressure- and volume-controlled models. They have separate air and oxygen supplies allowing accurate delivery of inspired oxygen concentration up to 100%.

illness (acute or chronic) and the aims of support at the time it is applied (e.g. delivery of IPPV or weaning). PEEP prevents the baseline airway pressure returning to atmospheric (0 cmH$_2$O on the ventilator manometer) at end-expiration. PEEP prevents alveolar collapse at end-expiration, increasing functional residual capacity and improving compliance. Recruitment of atelectatic alveoli is encouraged, and V/Q mismatch reduced.

Ventilation in specific clinical conditions
Patients with asthma or COPD

Severe expiratory airflow obstruction occurs in most patients with asthma and COPD who need invasive ventilation. Ventilatory management can be complicated by significant gas trapping. This increases intra-thoracic pressure (so-called auto-PEEP) and can lead to a reduction in venous return with a fall in cardiac output and acute hypotension. Successful ventilatory strategies involve deliberate hypoventilation with slow ventilator rates and reduced tidal volumes with a long expiratory time to allow for improved lung emptying. This successfully reduces mean airway pressure and barotrauma, but often results in hypercapnia, which is usually well tolerated.

Most patients who are ventilated for severe asthma, who do not suffer a pre-hospital cardiac arrest, will make a full recovery. Between 45% and 65% of patients ventilated with COPD survive critical care admission. However, many will be readmitted to hospital within 6 months of discharge with further exacerbations. Discussions with patients who have needed invasive ventilation are important to allow them to make informed decisions about their treatment preferences in future severe exacerbations.

Patients with acute lung injury/acute respiratory distress syndrome, the lung protection approach

Acute lung injury (ALI) and its extreme manifestation, the acute respiratory distress syndrome (ARDS), complicate a wide variety of serious medical and surgical conditions, not all of which affect the lung directly. ALI and ARDS are defined by varying degrees of refractory hypoxaemia seen in association with bilateral lung infiltrates on chest radiography, in the presence of a clinical condition known to precipitate the syndrome but in the absence of left atrial hypertension (thereby excluding hydrostatic pulmonary oedema as a cause) (Figure 7.8). The characteristic distribution of lung injury means regions that are relatively unaffected receive a disproportionate volume of the delivered breath. They are therefore at risk of overdistension (volutrauma) and, if the positive pressure is high, to barotrauma. Cyclical opening and closing of damaged lung are thought to generate pro-inflammatory mediators (biotrauma). To minimize these complications, low tidal volume ventilation (6 mL/kg body weight) is mandated and affords a mortality advantage when compared to traditional approaches (e.g. 10 mL/kg). This 'lung protection' approach can result in reduced clearance of carbon dioxide (CO_2) with resulting hypercapnia and respiratory acidosis. 'Permissive' hypercapnia is, however, an acceptable side effect provided oxygenation is not compromised and the pH is maintained above 7.2. The success of this approach has renewed interest in high frequency ventilation or

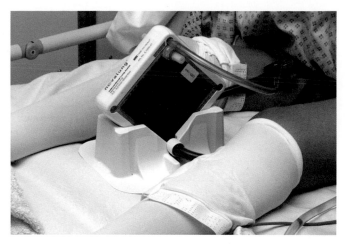

Figure 7.9 A Novolung device. This is one type of extra-corporeal gas exchanging device. A number of clinical trials are currently being performed with such devices in acute lung injury.

oscillation, in which small tidal volumes (less than anatomical deadspace) are administered at very high frequencies and gas exchange occurs by convection. As yet there is insufficient evidence to conclude whether high-frequency ventilation reduces mortality or long-term morbidity in patients with ALI or ARDS. A number of non-ventilatory adjuncts to gas exchange have been used in acute lung injury. These include high-dose steroids, prone positioning, inhaled nitric oxide and extracorporeal gas exchange (Figure 7.9). None of these interventions are currently supported by high-grade evidence but further clinical trials are in progress and they may be applied appropriately in individual patients as rescue therapy.

Weaning from mechanical ventilation

Prolonged mechanical ventilation is associated with increased morbidity and mortality and increases the risk of weaning failure. Weaning involves the gradual increase in the amount of time the patient is breathing spontaneously whilst the level of ventilatory support is gradually decreased. Modes of ventilation used in weaning include synchronized intermittent mandatory ventilation (SIMV), BiPAP, pressure support (assisted spontaneous breathing) and CPAP. In patients with COPD non-invasive ventilation can be used to continue weaning following extubation. This has been shown to reduce weaning time, shorten ICU length of stay, reduce nosocomial pneumonia and improve 60-day survival rates.

Further reading

ARDSNet Group. Ventilation with lower tidal volumes as compared with traditional tidal volumes for acute lung injury and the acute respiratory distress syndrome. The Acute Respiratory Distress Syndrome Network. *N Engl J Med* 2000; 342:1301–8.

Baudouin SV. Invasive mechanical ventilation. *Medicine* 2008; 36:250–2.

British Thoracic Society Standards of Care Committee. British Thoracic Society Guideline. Non-invasive ventilation in acute respiratory failure. *Thorax* 2002; 57:192–211.

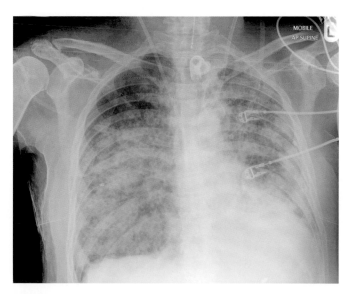

Figure 7.8 Plain radiograph from a patient with severe acute lung injury. Widespread bilateral airspace shadowing is present.

Griffiths J, Barber VS, Morgan L, Young JD. Systematic review and meta-analysis of studies of the timing of tracheostomy in adult patients undergoing artificial ventilation. *BMJ* 2005; 330:1243.

Leaver SK, Evans TW. Acute respiratory distress syndrome. *BMJ* 2007; 335:389–94.

Online tutorial

There is an online tutorial on this subject at http://www.scottish intensive-care.org.uk/education/index.htm. Click on the 'Induction tutorials' tab to find it.

CHAPTER 8

Cardiovascular Support

Neil Soni[1] *and David Watson*[2]

[1]Chelsea and Westminster Hospital, London, UK
[2]Barts and The London School of Medicine, London, UK

OVERVIEW

- Aim for an effective cardiac output (ECO) defined by warm perfused peripheries, normal blood pressure, reasonable pulse rate and evidence of satisfactory organ function
- A relationship exists between pressure, flow and resistance. Changing one variable will have an effect on the other two
- Identify the cause of the problem and match the intervention to the cause, for example mechanical problems are usually best fixed mechanically
- Concurrent maintenance of adequate oxygenation and haemoglobin level will help to achieve effective tissue oxygen delivery
- Cardiovascular support is required not only for hypotension or shock but also to prevent complications in patients at risk of organ failure

Cardiovascular physiology

The cardiovascular system is the main transport system of the body. Cardiovascular function can be affected at any part of the system (Figure 8.1). It is a hydraulic system and as such obeys physical principles. The equation $V = IR$ can be used where

V — pressure — blood pressure gradient
I = flow – cardiac output (CO)
R = resistance – peripheral resistance to outflow.

This is commonly represented as $MAP - CVP = CO \times SVR$, where MAP is mean arterial blood pressure; CVP is central venous pressure; SVR is systemic vascular resistance (the peripheral resistance to outflow).

If blood pressure falls it may be corrected by an increase in cardiac output or resistance or both. If cardiac output falls the blood pressure may be sustainable by an increase in peripheral vascular resistance. If resistance falls then blood pressure might be maintained if the cardiac output increases. Increases in peripheral

vascular resistance may result in either a rise in blood pressure or a fall in cardiac output (the former associated with an increase in cardiac work as blood pressure × cardiac output reflects cardiac work undertaken).

Cardiovascular malfunction

Any hydraulic system needs adequate fluid to fill the system, and an adequate working pressure to generate flow. An awareness of the normal responses to reduced cardiac output is helpful. These are largely mediated by pressure, volume and oxygen-sensitive receptors (Figure 8.2).

Failure of the cardiovascular system is called shock. This is defined as acute circulatory failure with inadequate or inappropriately distributed tissue perfusion resulting in cellular hypoxia. Shock can be classified as cardiogenic, obstructive, hypovolaemic or distributive shock but, in clinical practice, these commonly overlap (Box 8.1). For example, in sepsis vasodilatation and fluid sequestration leads to hypovolaemia (relative or absolute) and may also be associated with a reduction in myocardial contractility.

Box 8.1 **Types of shock**

- Cardiogenic shock: caused by 'pump failure', for example acute myocardial infarction
- Obstructive shock: caused by mechanical impediment to forward flow, for example, pulmonary embolus, cardiac tamponade, tension pneumothorax
- Hypovolaemic shock: caused by loss of circulating volume. These losses may be exogenous (haemorrhage, burns) or endogenous (through leaks in the microcirculation or into body cavities as occurs in intestinal obstruction)
- Distributive shock: caused by abnormalities of the peripheral circulation, for example, sepsis and anaphylaxis

Identifying tissue hypoperfusion

Clinical – Evaluate skin colour and temperature, capillary refill, pulse volume and sweating. There may be clinical evidence of poor organ perfusion such as altered conscious level, chest or abdominal pain, or oliguria.

ABC of Intensive Care, Second Edition.
Edited by Graham R. Nimmo and Mervyn Singer.

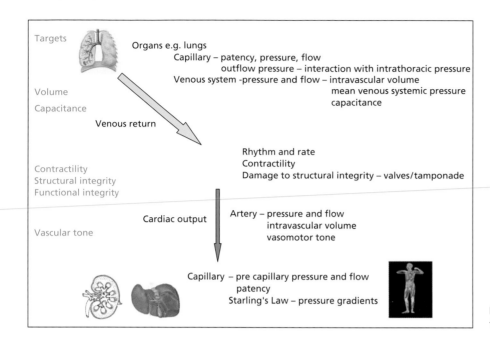

Figure 8.1 Factors that alter cardiovascular function. Targets for therapy are listed.

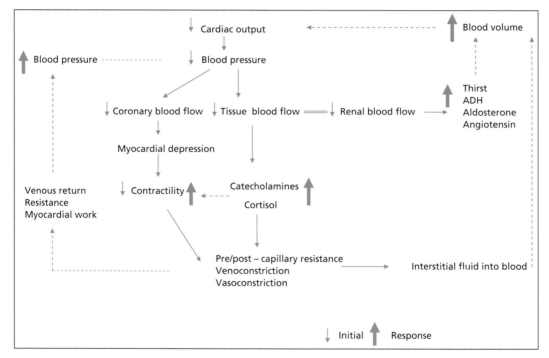

Figure 8.2 Assimilation of the key main effects following a fall in cardiac output. The arrows indicate the effects of falling output while the dotted lines indicate some of the main responses. Also shown are the targets for treatment.

Core – peripheral temperature gradient increases with hypo-volaemia or reduced perfusion (not a reliable guide to cardiac output or to peripheral resistance).

Metabolic acidosis with raised blood lactate concentration occurs if tissue perfusion is inadequate to meet metabolic needs so that cellular hypoxia and anaerobic glycolysis occurs.

All of these signs must be evaluated together and in the context of the clinical situation, as they may be misleading if interpreted in isolation.

Support goals

The first step is to identify the part of the system that is failing. It may be either the tone of the vascular system, inadequate intravascular volume and/or failing myocardial contractility. The cause should be sought and addressed and the particular physiological problem corrected. The fundamental aim of support is to provide an effective cardiac output (ECO), which is the composite of the elements of an intact cardiovascular system (Box 8.2). Clinical and physiological improvement in the features of hypoperfusion detailed above indicates that oxygen delivery is improving to meet metabolic demands. Functional response to organ support and treatment (FROST) is when an effective cardiac output has been achieved. This basic bedside clinical approach avoids specific focus on a measurement number such as cardiac output which, for any individual at any given time, is meaningless without the rest of the clinical context. This has been an issue in haemodynamic management as new technologies producing isolated numbers have in part replaced the more holistic clinical overview.

Box 8.2 A description of effective cardiac output (ECO)

- Warm well-perfused peripheries
- Blood pressure within acceptable range for the individual
- Pulse rate within acceptable range
- Evidence of functioning of organs, for example passing urine, normal mentation
- Clearance or absence of lactic acidosis

Target areas for diagnosis and treatment

The objective is to restore oxygen delivery to the tissues through ECO while correcting the underlying cause, for example surgical intervention to arrest haemorrhage or surgical drainage of an infected focus. Speed is essential.

Intravascular volume (preload)

Hydraulic systems require fluid to function. An adequate circulating blood volume is vital to a functional cardiovascular system. The reflex, protective consequences of hypovolaemia include peripheral vasoconstriction intended to divert blood supply to central vital organs such as heart, lungs and brain. To improve perfusion to less vital areas the system must be refilled by volume resuscitation (Box 8.3), which results in a slow reduction in vasoconstriction. In Figure 8.3 the difficulties of using pressures (such as central venous pressure) to indicate volume are demonstrated. Pressure does not equate to volume and hence 'filling pressures' are misleading unless taken in the context of peripheral perfusion. The heart needs an adequate venous return and so an adequate intravascular volume is fundamental to cardiovascular performance. The Frank–Starling curve shows increasing cardiac output as venous return increases (Figure 8.4).

Box 8.3 Choice of fluid for volume replacement

- *Blood*: Clearly indicated in haemorrhagic shock and to maintain the haemoglobin concentration at an acceptable level (conventionally > 70 g/L or packed cell volume > 30%) in shock due to other causes
- *Crystalloids*: Cheap, convenient to use, and free of side-effects but rapidly distributed across the intravascular and interstitial spaces; volumes 1.5 times that of colloid are required to achieve an equivalent haemodynamic response. Volume expansion is more transient, more fluid may accumulate in the interstitial spaces and pulmonary oedema may result

---

- *Colloids*: (albumin, gelatins, hetastarches) produce a more sustained increase in plasma volume with associated improvements in cardiovascular function and oxygen transport though carry their own potential side-effects such as coagulopathy and anaphylactoid reactions

---

The heart

The heart is a pump that needs an adequate blood volume and venous return, a functional anatomy, and to work at an optimal rate and with an intact hydraulic system.

Functional structure

Forward flow requires functional one-way valves. Both valvular regurgitation and stenosis impede forward flow. Ventricular wall

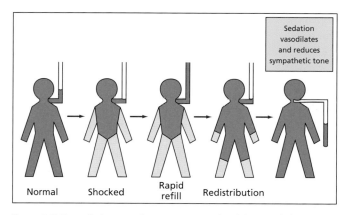

Sedation vasodilates and reduces sympathetic tone

Normal   Shocked   Rapid refill   Redistribution

Figure 8.3 Normal: the central venous pressure (CVP) is normal, the patient is 'full'. (b) The patient loses blood, becomes shocked (white areas), the CVP is low. (c) Rapid refill: if patients are given fluid rapidly they may still be vasoconstricted and so the CVP rises yet the intravascular volume is still low. (d) Redistribution as vasodilation takes place. The CVP falls, demonstrating the patient's true volume status. If the patient markedly vasodilates, as might happen if sedated and sympathetic tone is lost, hypotension may ensue as the patient is effectively hypovolaemic and now has a low CVP.

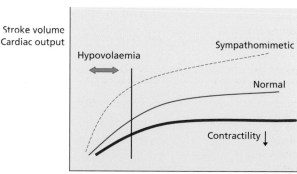

Stroke volume / Cardiac output

Hypovolaemia

Sympathomimetic

Normal

Contractility ↓

Preoad/venous return/end diastolic volume/atrial filling pressure/ cvp

Figure 8.4 Frank–Starling curve. A reduced preload reduces cardiac output. As the preload or ventricular filling increases, the cardiac output also rises. In the failing heart with impaired contractility the effect is depressed. Catecholamines increase contractility and enhance this effect.

size may also alter ventricular capacity. External constriction or pressure caused by pathology such as pericardial tamponade or tension pneumothorax will prevent cardiac filling and diminish cardiac output. Outflow obstruction, such as pulmonary embolus, also reduces cardiac output.

Cardiac rate and rhythm

These are important factors in maintaining an adequate cardiac output. Ventricular filling is time dependent and significantly aided by atrial contraction. Increased ventricular rate may compromise chamber filling as does loss of atrial contraction, thereby impairing cardiac performance. Slowing of the heart will functionally reduce the amount of blood being expelled over a period of time and hence reduce cardiac output. However, slowing a tachycardia may allow more efficient filling and a more effective ventricle, while speeding up a slow heart will also increase overall cardiac output. In the critically ill patient tachyarrhythmias such as atrial fibrillation are common. Digoxin, amiodarone and beta-blockade can be used to control rate. Digoxin, a time-honoured drug, may also benefit contractility. Amiodarone is effective for rate control and has a mild vasodilatory action which may reduce myocardial work in the failing ventricle.

Cardiac contractility

This is affected not only by damage, ischaemia or infarction (Figure 8.5) but also by the altered geometry of the heart if part of the ventricular wall is moving abnormally. Inadequate contractility decreases cardiac output and almost invariably reduces efficiency thus cardiac workload is relatively increased to maintain output. This may further compromise the ventricle, especially if ischaemic.

Inotropes (Table 8.1)

The endogenous catecholamines adrenaline, noradrenaline and dopamine usually increase cardiac contractility and hence increase blood pressure. There are variable effects on the vasculature. At low dose, both adrenaline and dopamine causes some vasodilation (beta-adrenoreceptor mediated) but vasoconstrict at higher doses (alpha-adrenoreceptor mediated). Noradrenaline produces mainly vasoconstriction.

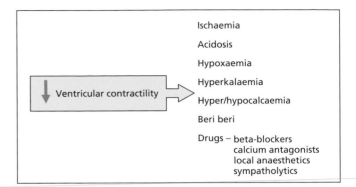

Figure 8.5 Causes of decreased ventricular contractility.

Dopamine, a drug currently out of favour, is an effective inotrope with a gentle dose–response contractility curve, vasodilator properties at low and vasoconstrictor actions at higher dose. Dopaminergic effects are hard to demonstrate in clinical situations, although the agent can cause a natriuresis. Inotropes that vasodilate are popular in managing the failing heart where constrictors increase myocardial work. The concept of increasing contractility while simultaneously reducing outflow resistance or afterload is ideal, provided blood pressure is not unduly compromised. Dobutamine, dopexamine and phosphodiesterase inhibitors (enoximone, milrinone) are inotropes with vasodilatory actions that may be effective in the failing heart. However, the vasodilatation will unmask any covert hypovolaemia as demonstrated by potentially severe hypotension. Rapid infusion of intravenous fluids should be commenced in this situation with pressor agents occasionally being needed to counter the hypotensive effect. The new agent levisomendan is probably best described as a calcium sensitizing drug that does not increase intracellular calcium but does increase contractility. It is also a vasodilator with potential utility in cardiac failure. There is also interest in its cautious use in sepsis.

The role of beta-blockers in heart failure is changing. Traditionally, the negative inotropic effects of these drugs militated against their use in the critically ill and this is still a major consideration. However, as they reduce cardiac workload and hence myocardial oxygen requirements, they may be protective. They are also effective in hypertensive heart failure as cardiac work is reduced through blood pressure lowering.

Table 8.1 Receptor actions of sympathomimetic and dopaminergic drugs.

	β_1	β_2	α_1	α_2	DA$_1$	DA$_2$
Adrenaline						
Low dose	+	+	+	±	NA	NA
High dose	++(+)	++(+)	++++	+++	NA	NA
Noradrenaline	++	0	+++	+++	NA	NA
Isoprenaline	+++	+++	0	0	NA	NA
Dopamine						
Moderate dose	++	+	++	+	++(+)	+
High dose	+++	++	+++	+	++(+)	+
Dopexamine	+	+++	0	0	++	+
Dobutamine	++	+	±	?	0	0

NA, not applicable.

The tone of the vasculature (afterload) affects cardiac function

Arterial vasodilation (afterload reduction) reduces myocardial work to achieve a given output, hence vasodilators or inodilators may prove very effective in cardiac failure. The risk is relative hypotension and achieving a balance where both pressure and flow are adequate is the goal. Arterial vasoconstriction will increase blood pressure though at the expense of increased ventricular work. In practice, a balance is sought to produce an adequate cardiac output with an acceptable blood pressure by manipulating both cardiac contractility and vasomotor tone. In severe sepsis, profound vasodilation is associated with a high cardiac output (even with impaired cardiac contractility) and is often accompanied by a compromised blood pressure ('septic shock'). Low diastolic pressures may further impair coronary artery filling and alter myocardial contractility through secondary ischaemia. Vasoconstrictor and inotropic support may both be required to maintain an effective blood flow and blood pressure. The interaction between heart and vasculature means that neither should ever be considered in isolation. Perfusion, pressure and organ function is the combined goal. (Figure 8.6).

Constrictors

Catecholamines at high dose, in particular noradrenaline, are potent vasoconstrictors. Phenylephrine is a selective α_1-agonist that vasoconstricts in isolation, hence may be useful when vasodilation is the primary problem after hypovolaemia has been corrected. However, the blood pressure rise is usually impressive but unpredictable between individuals and may result in reflex bradycardia. Furthermore, the increase in cardiac workload imposed by the high resistance can be catastrophic in a failing ventricle. Vasopressin is a potent vasoconstrictor acting via vasopressinergic receptors. It is used in septic and other types of vasodilatory shock but is not innocuous and can induce coronary, mesenteric or digital ischaemia.

Dilators

Dilating the vascular system reduces outflow resistance (afterload), reducing cardiac work and improving cardiac output. The increase in venous capacitance will tend to reduce venous return, which may necessitate fluid administration. While extremely useful in conditions with fluid overload or a failing ventricle, these agents may cause profound falls in blood pressure if there is covert hypovolaemia. In acute circumstances glyceryl trinitrate and sodium nitroprusside can be used to control high blood pressure or to improve cardiac output from a failing heart. Glyceryl trinitrate is a potent vasodilator that acts through release of either nitric oxide or a closely related species. It can be given sublingually, orally or by skin patch; however, in the critically ill, it is ideally suited for administration by continuous intravenous infusion. It acts on venous capacitance vessels but also has marked arterial dilating effects, particular at higher doses. As such it is a 'user-friendly' agent in the critically ill and may assist in improving capillary perfusion.

Sodium nitroprusside is a very potent non-selective vasodilator with rapid onset and offset of action on both arterial and venous vessels. It will reduce arterial tone rapidly but will also increase venous capacitance, thereby reducing venous return. All of the above will influence cardiac output. It can be toxic if dosage limitations are exceeded and is not a first-line drug except where hypertension is immediately life threatening.

In the longer term, oral vasodilators such as angiotensin-converting enzyme (ACE) inhibitors and calcium antagonists are used for blood pressure control.

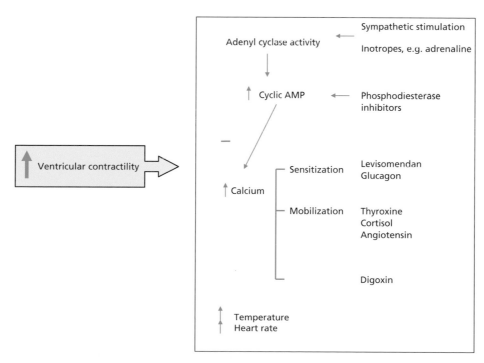

Figure 8.6 Mechanisms to increase ventricular contractility.

Mechanical interventions

Cardiac pacing

Cardiac pacing is indicated if the heart rate is too slow and proves refractory to chronotropic drug administration, for example atropine, isoproterenol, salbutamol or adrenaline. Pacemakers are increasingly versatile. Atrioventricular pacing can improve myocardial filling and hence contraction, or it can be used to control inefficient rhythms.

Continuous positive airway pressure and intermittent positive pressure ventilation

CPAP and IPPV have a role in the patient with the failing ventricle. Improved oxygenation, reduction in the work of breathing, redistribution of pulmonary oedema, reduced cardiac work (through offloading of the right ventricle and reduced afterload to the left ventricle) and an increased gradient between intrathoracic and extrathoracic compartments all augment left ventricular function and the oxygen supply–demand balance.

The intra-aortic counterpulsation balloon pump augments the aortic diastolic pressure, aids coronary perfusion and reduces afterload by balloon deflation during systole. It can be used to support a failing ventricle while definitive management is sought or while the ventricle recovers.

Left ventricular assist devices in specialist centres can be also be used in an attempt to preserve ventricular function while definitive treatment is sought.

Further reading

Chatti R, Fradj NB, Trabelsi W, *et al*. Algorithm for therapeutic management of acute heart failure syndromes. *Heart Fail Rev* 2007; 12:113–7.

Improving Surgical Outcomes Group www.ebpom.org.

Resuscitation Council www.resus.org.uk

Rudiger A, Singer M. Mechanisms of sepsis-induced cardiac dysfunction. *Crit Care Med* 2007; 35:1599–608.

The Surviving Sepsis Campaign www. survivingsepsis.org

CHAPTER 9

Renal Failure

Liam Plant[1] and Alasdair Short[2]

[1]Department of Renal Medicine, Cork University Hospital, Cork, Ireland
[2]Broomfield Hospital, Chelmsford, UK

OVERVIEW

- A standardised system for definition and stratification for acute kidney injury (AKI) should be adopted
- All cases of AKI need (i) evaluation of extracellular fluid/intravascular volume status, (ii) evaluation of systemic cardiovascular performance, (iii) review of medications, (iv) reagent strip urinalysis and (v) renal tract sonography
- Generic management of associated clinical problems is the mainstay of management for most cases of AKI
- There is no evidence base to support the use of any specific pharmaceutical agent in the prevention or treatment of AKI
- Renal replacement therapies should reflect local competencies; optimal dosage is subject to a number of ongoing trials

---

AKI (also known as acute renal failure) is a clinical syndrome characterised by rapid deterioration in the excretory and other functions of the kidneys (Box 9.1 and Table 9.1). It is commonly encountered in intensive care, particularly as an element of the multi-organ dysfunction syndrome (MODS). Development of AKI, even to degrees previously considered as 'mild', is associated with a substantial increase in morbidity and mortality, complexity of care and resource consumption. Some cases will require treatment with renal replacement therapy (RRT), usually haemofiltration or haemodialysis. Although most cases of AKI can be successfully managed by intensive care physicians, the range and potential complexity of cases requires ongoing consultation with the local nephrology service. Many of these patients will have pre-existing chronic kidney disease (CKD), some will not fully recover from AKI, and patients will need to transition from the ICU/HDU environment to a general ward setting. For all of these scenarios, nephrological input is appropriate. Local guidelines should be in place to facilitate this.

Box 9.1 **Functions of the kidney**

Homeostasis

- Maintenance of fluid balance
- Regulation of sodium, potassium, phosphate concentrations

- Excretion of metabolic waste products: urea, creatinine, ammonia, uric acid
- Maintenance of normal acid-base balance
- Drug and toxin metabolism and elimination

Hormonal

- Erythropoietin production
- Vitamin D and calcium metabolism: activation of 25-OH-cholecalciferol
- Renin–angiotensin system

Definition and staging systems

Systematic evaluation of the incidence, severity and outcome of AKI has been previously hampered by a multitude of definitions and stratification systems. A uniform definition and multilevel stratification has been proposed by the Acute Kidney Injury Network (AKIN), an international consensus group of critical care physicians and nephrologists. The AKIN system developed from the 2004 Risk/Insult/Failure/Loss/End stage kidney disease (RIFLE) proposal of the Acute Dialysis Quality Initiative group.

Many parameters are disturbed in AKI. The presence of *either* of two specific criteria allows definition and stratification. These are:

- absolute or relative increments in serum [creatinine]
- reduced urine volume.

Table 9.1 Acute Kidney Injury Network (AKIN) staging system for acute kidney injury.

AKIN stage	Increment in serum [creatinine]	Urine output
1	Absolute increase ≥26.4 μmol/L or Increase to 150–199% of baseline	<0.5 mL/kg/h for >6 h
2	Increase to 200–299% of baseline	<0.5 mL/kg/h for >12 h
3	Absolute value ≥354 μmol/L (provided increase ≥44 μmol/L) or Increase to 300% of baseline or institution of renal replacement therapy	<0.3 ml/kg/h for >24 h or anuric for >12 h

ABC of Intensive Care, Second Edition.
Edited by Graham R. Nimmo and Mervyn Singer.
© 2011 Blackwell Publishing Ltd. Published 2011 by Blackwell Publishing Ltd.

Table 9.2 Domains of causes of acute kidney injury.

Pre-renal	Renal	Post-renal
Hypovolaemia (diarrhoea, vomiting, excessive diuresis, fluid sequestration)	Glomerulonephritis	Luminal obstruction (kidney stones, drug precipitation)
	Microscopic polyarteritis (Goodpasture syndrome, Wegener's granulomatosis, SLE)	Intrinsic obstruction (urothelial malignancy)
Hypotension (haemorrhagic cardiogenic, septic shock; tachy- and bradydysrhythmias, pericardial effusion)	Accelerated hypertension	Extrinsic obstruction (prostatic disease, cervical and ovarian malignancies, retroperitoneal fibrosis)
	Athero-embolisation	
Drugs disrupting intra-renal perfusion (NSAIDs, radiocontrast agents, ACEi's)	Pigment induced (rhabdomyolysis)	
	Myeloma cast nephropathy	
	Interstitial nephritis (antibiotics, NSAIDs)	
Hepatorenal syndrome	Thrombotic thrombocytopenic purpura	
	Acute tubular necrosis	

ACEi, angiotension-converting enzyme inhibitors; NSAIDs, non-steroidal anti-inflammatory drugs, SLE, systemic lupus erythematosus.

The timescale for observation is over a 48-hour period. The highest stage attained is an important predictor of outcome.

Causes of acute kidney injury

The traditional classification of AKI describes pre-renal, renal (parenchymal), and post-renal causes (Table 9.2). There is considerable overlap between these.

The commonest cause (50–75%) of impaired renal function is pre-renal AKI, usually as a result of shock.

The first step in the production of urine is glomerular filtration. This is dependent upon both systemic cardiovascular function and intra-renal haemodynamics, which under normal circumstances are tightly controlled to generate an intra-glomerular filtration pressure, resulting in appropriate glomerular filtration rate (GFR). The energy consumption for this process is entirely extra-renal. Decreased renal perfusion leads to a continuum extending from a rapidly volume/perfusion pressure-responsive decline in GFR to (potentially recoverable) histological changes of acute tubular necrosis (ATN). Pre-existing chronic kidney disease (CKD), heart failure, liver disease, increasing age and co-administration of medications interfering with intra-renal haemodynamics (e.g. non-steroidal anti-inflammatories, COX-2 inhibitors, angiotensin-converting enzyme (ACE) inhibitors) increase the sensitivity of the kidneys to such ischaemic insults, as does the presence of sepsis and the systemic inflammatory response syndrome (SIRS).

Intrinsic AKI involves (potentially reversible) structural damage to glomeruli, tubules, vessels and interstitium. This may result from pre-renal AKI with the development of ATN, or reflect idiosyncratic or dose-dependent drug toxicity. Immunologically mediated causes

such as interstitial nephritis or glomerulonephritis are uncommon, which sometimes means that they are overlooked in the diagnostic workup, resulting in delay in diagnosis and irreversible loss of renal function (many of these processes result in non-reversible scarring). Post-renal causes include any kind of obstruction of tubules, ureters or bladder.

Epidemiology and outcomes

In the UK, annual incidence of AKI is 450–650 cases per million population, with up to 200 cases per million requiring RRT. It is more commonly acquired in hospital (7% of admissions) than in the community (1% of admissions). Approximately 35–50% of patients have pre-existing CKD. Of critically ill patients managed in the ICU, 10–62% develop AKI and 3–5% receive RRT. Nearly 10% of ICU beds are occupied by patients with AKI. Illustrative data are presented in Figure 9.1.

Up to 50% of patients developing AKIN stage 1 (RIFLE-RISK) progress to a higher stage. Hospital stay and in-hospital mortality is greater in these patients than in those who remain in stage 1 or who do not develop AKI.

AKI itself probably independently contributes to mortality; however, outcomes also depend upon illness severity (measured as APACHE-II score) at admission, failure of other organs, and the patient's age and comorbidity profile. In those who have developed AKI in addition to their primary condition, mortality at 60 days and at 6 months is significantly increased. End-stage kidney disease (irreversible renal failure) is much less common. If only the kidney has failed, mortalities of up to 10% are expected. This rises to> 50% in multi-organ failure.

Sixty-five per cent to 85% of survivors recover renal function and become independent of RRT. This variation is related to cause and underlying comorbidity.

Diagnosis and evaluation

Patients should be evaluated early in the course of their illness. The core evaluation should consist of the following.

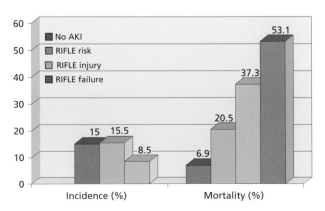

Figure 9.1 Incidence of different stages (RIFLE staging) of acute kidney injury with corresponding mortality.

Patient history with especial focus on pre-existing CKD, heart failure and liver disease
Drug history with particular focus on exposure to nephrotoxic agents
Clinical evaluation for evidence of cardiovascular dysfunction/sepsis
Evaluation of extracellular fluid (ECF) volume status (with central venous pressure monitoring as indicated)
Reagent strip urinalysis (with urine microscopy as indicated)
Ultrasound scanning of urinary tract morphology (to exclude obstruction and to assess kidney size) is mandatory

A decline in urine output is a very sensitive, but not specific, early sign that AKI may be developing and often occurs before changes in serum [creatinine]. Urine output may not be accurately measured outside the critical care environment. Its interpretation depends upon the clinical context (patient may be obstructed or have uncorrected extra-cellular fluid (ECF) volume depletion or another cause of hypotension).

A variety of derived indices utilising urinary biochemistry are traditionally employed in the evaluation of AKI. There is little systematic evidence to support their utility, especially in patients with AKI due to sepsis. Measuring eGFR is of no value in the non-steady state of AKI.

Many studies have evaluated the use of new biomarkers such as cystatin-C, kidney injury molecule (KIM-1) and neutrophil gelatinase-associated lipocalin (NGAL). These seem to be superior predictors of AKI (but not requirement for RRT nor potential for recovery) than serum [creatinine], but their place in normal clinical practice is still to be established.

Haematuria and/or proteinuria should prompt evaluation for glomerular or interstitial disease. This may involve testing for:

- anti-glomerular basement membrane antibodies (aGBM)
- anti-neutrophil cytoplasmic antibodies (ANCA)
- anti-nuclear antibodies (ANF)
- serum immunoglobulins and electrophoresis
- complement levels.

Under these circumstances early specialist nephrological input is essential and some patients will require a renal biopsy.

Generic management

The kidney is an organ with considerable capacity both to protect itself from and to recover from damage. Cases encountered in the ICU predominantly belong to the volume-responsive AKI/hypotension/septic shock/ATN continuum. Excellence in resuscitation and correction/management of underlying problems such as sepsis, cardiovascular dysfunction or surgical problems are central to management.

The principles of generic management are:

- correction of hypoxaemia
- correction of ECF volume depletion and maintenance of an appropriate haemoglobin level

- restoration of adequate perfusion pressure
- correction of underlying clinical problems
- withdrawal and avoidance of nephrotoxins.

Careful clinical assessment, supplemented, as appropriate, by measurement of intra-arterial pressure, central venous pressure, cardiac output and urine output should guide resuscitation. Large volumes of crystalloids or physiologically unbalanced colloids may lead to further acid–base or electrolyte disturbances. On their own they often fail to restore perfusion pressure adequately in the presence of sepsis/SIRS or drugs that paralyse normal vasoconstrictive responses (e.g. ACE inhibitors). Under these circumstances vasopressors (e.g. noradrenaline) will be required after adequate fluid resuscitation. These should be administered in an appropriate critical care setting. Large volumes of 10% hetastarch solution may be associated with an increased risk of AKI. Hyperkalaemia may be a risk with use of Ringer's lactate or Hartmann's solutions.

Obstruction of the urinary tract, if present, should be corrected or bypassed. In a minority of cases involving glomerular disease or interstitial disease a decision as to the need for immunosuppressive therapy may be necessary.

In AKI, the pharmacokinetics of many drugs are altered and appropriate adjustments in prescription and dosage are necessary. Contrast-mediated nephropathy is also more likely and can be minimised by maintaining adequate ECF volume expansion, possibly supplemented by the use of N-acetylcysteine (NAC) combined with sodium bicarbonate administration.

Specific pharmacological therapies

As a general principle, there is no compelling evidence of benefit from any specific pharmacological agent. Despite continued use of loop diuretics, dopamine and mannitol as specific therapies for AKI, no adequately powered prospective study or meta-analysis has ever demonstrated benefit in terms of length of hospitalisation, requirement for RRT, duration of RRT, renal recovery or survival. All of these agents have significant side-effects and in the absence of any evidence of benefit should be avoided for specific treatment or prevention of acute renal impairment. The same applies to atrial natriuretic peptide. Studies on the possible utility of fenoldopam are ongoing. Growth factors such as insulin-like growth factor-1 have theoretical potential to speed up recovery from AKI; however, this has yet to be confirmed in clinical practice.

Renal replacement therapy

The decision to initiate RRT should be based on clinical parameters such as ECF volume status, electrolyte levels and metabolic state. Certain levels of severity provide 'traditional' indications for RRT. These include pulmonary oedema, hyperkalaemia resistant to non-RRT management, pericarditis, severe azotaemia and metabolic acidosis. However, if it is evident that resuscitation or other specific treatments are unlikely to lead to a rapid recovery of renal function, then early initiation of RRT is recommended, particularly in the context of multi-organ failure.

Renal replacement modality

A range of extracorporeal RRT modalities are available (Table 9.3). Peritoneal dialysis is also possible but, outwith paediatric practice, this is not commonly used in the ICU treatment of AKI.

When comparing modalities, the important issues are the efficiency of removal of small and middle sized solutes; the ease with which salt and water control can be achieved; and how well the patient tolerates the regimen. In addition, most systems will require some anticoagulation of the extra-corporeal circuit. Local competencies and equipment are the predominant factors informing choice of modality. With care, most modalities can be applied to any patient (even those with considerable haemodynamic instability), but the typical comparison between modalities is given in Table 9.4.

There has been a bias towards continuous (CRRT) rather than intermittent (iRRT) therapies in patients with greater cardiovascular instability. The Beginning Ending renal Support Therapy (BEST) group identified that over 80% of patients in a worldwide observational study were initially treated with CRRT. Prospective studies do not sustain the view that this improves outcome. There are no compelling studies showing an advantage in patient survival between iRRT and CRRT when corrected for comorbidities. Recovery of renal function (especially in those with more marked haemodynamic instability) may be higher if CRRT is used.

Dose of renal replacement therapy

Studies on urea kinetics can and should be used to quantify the 'intensity' of RRT treatments. For CRRT, it has been suggested that better outcomes are achieved with a haemofiltrate effluent of at least 35 mL/kg/hour. The BEST study however identified that only 11.7% of treatments actually achieve this; the median

delivered dose was 20.4 mL/kg/hour. The recent multicentre ATN study comparing effluent flows of 40 vs 25 mL/kg/hour showed no convincing evidence in support of more 'intensive' regimens.

It is important to recognise that prescribed and delivered therapy doses can be very different. In order to achieve a continuous haemofiltrate effluent of at least 20 mL/kg/hour a higher dose should be prescribed to allow for clotting/other interruptions in delivery. Prescriptions for iHD need to be on a daily or alternate day basis, with a delivered eKt/Vurea of 1.2 per treatment (this is a method of assessing dialysis dose based upon dialyser clearance K; time of treatment t, and total body water estimate V).

Access and anticoagulation

A sufficiently large access catheter is required for RRT. Central venous access is preferred and the internal jugular or common femoral veins are the favoured sites. The site should be carefully managed and lines changed appropriately to minimise the risk of infection. Complications associated with these lines include bleeding, pneumothorax, air embolism, sepsis and, in the longer term, central venous stenosis.

Patients with AKI are commonly hypercoagulable. This, in conjunction with the consequences of non-laminar blood flow though the extra-corporeal circuit, an air–blood interface, a membrane–blood interface and haemoconcentration, makes some form of anticoagulation necessary. Clotting of the extra-corporeal circuit compromises small solute clearances and control of ECF volume. However, anticoagulation can lead to bleeding complications, especially in septic patients.

The commonest agent used is unfractionated heparin (UFH). This is monitored by activated clotting time (ACT) or activated partial thromboplastin time (APTT) monitoring. Bleeding and heparin-induced thrombocytopenia are potential hazards. Low molecular weight heparins (LMWHs) offer little advantage and are much more difficult to monitor. Epoprostenol is used in patients perceived to be at higher risk of bleeding. Less commonly used are hirudin, nafamostat and argat.

Other techniques, such as 'no heparin/saline flush' methods, maintaining high blood flow rates and utilizing pre-filter fluid replacement reduce the risk of clotting. Regional citrate anticoagulation is gaining popularity as the technique associated with the fewest bleeding complications, but requires a more complex extracorporeal circuit and is more difficult to combine with CVVH alone. New techniques for the use of citrate are currently being introduced

Table 9.3 Types of extracorporeal renal replacement therapy modalities.

	Intermittent	Continuous
Diffusive	Haemodialysis (iHD)	Slow low efficiency dialysis (SLED)
Convective	Haemofiltration (iHF)	Continuous venovenous haemofiltration (CVVH)
		Continuous arteriovenous haemofiltration (CAVH)
Hybrid	Haemodiafiltration (iHDF)	Continuous venovenous haemodiafiltration (CVVHDF)
		Continuous arteriovenous haemodiafiltration (CAVHDF)

Table 9.4 Comparisons between renal replacement therapy modalities.

	Small solute clearance	ECF volume control	Anti-coagulation	Haemodynamically unstable patients
iHD	High	Moderate	Can avoid	Tolerate poorly
CVVH	Moderate	High	Can avoid	Tolerate well
Hybrid	High	High	Can avoid	Tolerate well
PD	Moderate	Moderate	No	Tolerate well

ECF; extracellular fluid; PD, peritoneal dialysis.

Nutrition

AKI is a pro-inflammatory state with a constellation of metabolic, immunological and nutritional disturbances. Patients commonly have concurrent illnesses. Certain RRT modalities, notably high-volume CVVH, are associated with losses of water-soluble substances such as amino acids, protein, trace elements such as selenium and water-soluble vitamins. In the critically ill patient enteral nutrition is the preferred modality and should ideally provide 20–35 kcal/kg/day and 1.5–1.7 g/kg/day of amino acids, particularly in hypercatabolic patients. Micronutrient supplementation is obligatory. In distinction to the problems occurring with management which do not include RRT, hypokalaemia and hypophosphataemia are potential issues with CRRT.

Further reading

Hoste EA, Lamiere NH, Vanholder RC, *et al*. Acute renal failure in patients with sepsis in a surgical ICU: predictive factors, incidence, comorbidity, and outcome. *J Am Soc Nephrol* 2003; 14:1022–30.

Joannidis M, Druml W, Forni LG, *et al*.; Critical Care Nephrology Working Group of the European Society of Intensive Care Medicine Prevention of acute kidney injury and protection of renal function in the intensive care unit. Expert opinion of the Working Group for Nephrology, ESICM. *Intensive Care Med* 2010; 36:392–411.

Mehta RL, Kellum JA, Shah SV, *et al*.; Acute Kidney Injury Network. Acute Kidney Injury Network: report of an initiative to improve outcomes in acute kidney injury. *Crit Care* 2007; 11:R31.

Renal Association. *Treatment of adults and children with renal failure: clinical practice guidelines and audit measures*, 4th edn. London: Royal College of Physicians of London and the Renal Association, 2008. www.renal.org/guidelines/module5.html.

Ricci Z, Ronco C. Kidney disease beyond nephrology: intensive care. *Nephrol Dial Transplant* 2008; 23:1–7.

VA/NIH Acute Renal Failure Trial Network. Intensity of renal support in critically ill patients with acute kidney injury. *N Engl J Med* 2008; 359:7–20.

Online tutorial

There is an online tutorial on this subject at http://www.scottish intensive-care.org.uk/education/index.htm. Click on the 'Induction tutorials' tab to find it.

CHAPTER 10

Neurological Support

Peter J. D. Andrews

Western General Hospital, Lothian University Hospitals Division, Edinburgh, UK

OVERVIEW

- Neurological critical care describes the coordinated efforts of many specialists, including intensive care experts, neurologists, neurosurgeons, anaesthetists, neuroradiologists, physiotherapists, specialist nurses and many others

- In common with all severely ill patients, emergency treatment must start with 'A.B.C.D.E.' management before any further investigation or procedure

- Coma is one of the most common problems encountered in intensive care medicine and accounts for a substantial proportion of admissions

- Management guidelines emphasize admission of all 'salvageable' head injury patients to a specialist centre, as this is associated with better outcomes

- It is important to implement therapies for which there is robust evidence, to avoid harmful interventions and to further investigate established strategies that lack evidence

Introduction

Neurological critical care describes the coordinated efforts of many specialists, including intensive care experts, neurologists, neurosurgeons, anaesthetists, neuroradiologists, physiotherapists, specialist nurses and many others. Specialized neurological monitoring and neurological imaging techniques (magnetic resonance imaging (MRI) and computed tomography (CT)) must also be available 24/7. The Neurological critical care unit (NCCU) serves as the focal point for these combined efforts.

History

Components of neurological critical care can be traced as far back as the days of trephination, fits and contagion. However, as the field of medical critical care developed, neurologists gradually withdrew from general critical care and neurology became chiefly a diagnostic discipline.

ABC of Intensive Care, Second Edition.
Edited by Graham R. Nimmo and Mervyn Singer.
© 2011 Blackwell Publishing Ltd. Published 2011 by Blackwell Publishing Ltd.

With the advent of thrombolytic treatment of stroke, there has been an increased interest in the management of ischaemic stroke, with the sequelae of reperfusion and haemorrhage. Neurologists and stroke physicians have become more 'interventional' as a result. However, as described below, there is an increasing need for neurological intensivists to be the primary physicians for these patients.

General principles

A diverse range of neurological conditions require management in the NCCU. Indications for admission are also varied, ranging from airway maintenance to seizure and intra-cranial pressure (ICP) control. Notwithstanding the wide range of neurological diseases, it is possible to describe a number of principles of intensive care management (Table 10.1).

In common with all severely ill patients, emergency treatment must start with A.B.C.D.E. management before further investigations or procedures are organized. Airway management is of utmost importance and the decision to intubate or not is sometimes a difficult one to make. Although the classic indication is a Glasgow Coma Score (GCS) of less than 9, some causes of coma are more easily and readily treatable, such as hypoglycaemia, seizures or some drug intoxication, and do not require intubation but close surveillance. On the other hand, in patients with large intra-axial haematoma(s), a large cerebellar infarct or severe brainstem damage, the patient should be intubated before the GCS decreases further and the airway is compromised. Cervical spine stabilization should be added whenever there is possibility of cervical trauma (even if there is no traumatic brain injury) or instability caused by medical disease, such as rheumatoid arthritis.

Mechanical ventilation management should maintain PaO_2 at approximately 100 mmHg (12 kPa) and $PaCO_2$ between 35 and 45 mmHg (4.5–6 kPa). Most patients require sedation to achieve these targets and although exclusion of sedatives is theoretically better for neurological observation, adequate gas exchange cannot be guaranteed with spontaneous ventilation.

The circulation must be maintained so that the brain receives adequate oxygen and substrates, and hypotension must be treated to maintain arterial blood pressure and thus cerebral perfusion pressure.

Table 10.1 General principles.

ICU management	Problem	Cause
Airway control (intubation/tracheostomy)	Loss of airway control	Decreased conscious level Brainstem dysfunction Neuropathy: cranial nerves : peripheral nerves
Mechanical ventilation	Respiratory failure	Decreased conscious level Brainstem dysfunction Neuropathy/neuromuscular/muscular disorder
Haemodynamic monitoring and support	Tachycardia, bradycardia Hypo-, hypertension, neurogenic pulm. oedema Inadequate CPP, requiring BP elevation	Autonomic neuropathy Subarachnoid haemorrhage Acute brain injury
ICP Mx and Rx	Raised ICP due to: Cerebral oedema Ischaemia/infarct Haemorrhage Hydrocephalus	Head injury Stroke Subarachnoid haemorrhage Encephalitis
EEG Mx and seizure control	Status epilepticus	Acute brain injury, encephalitis etc
Control of hyperirritability		Acute brain injury, encephalitis
Special procedures	IVIg infusion, thrombolysis	Guillain–Barré syndrome, Stroke Myasthenia gravis

EEG, electroencephalogram; ICP, intra-cranial pressure.

In the emergency situation initial management of comatose patients includes administration of intravenous glucose (25 g) unless blood testing can immediately exclude hypoglycaemia. Pre-morbid nutritional depletion may lead to Wernicke's encephalopathy with mental confusion; therefore thiamine, a co-factor for several enzymes supporting energy metabolism, should be given in all cases of coma before carbohydrate administration.

It is important to consider specific reversal agents or antagonists like naloxone (0.4–2 mg) for narcotic drug overdose, or flumazenil in the case of excess benzodiazepines. Such antidotes must be used with great care since they may produce an acute withdrawal syndrome in an addicted patient or seizures in susceptible patients.

Glasgow Coma Scale (and Score)

The GCS provides a framework for describing the state of a patient in terms of three aspects of responsiveness: eye opening, verbal response and best motor response, each stratified according to increasing impairment. The Glasgow Coma Scale Score (GCSS) is an artificial index, obtained by adding scores for the three responses. This score can provide a useful single figure summary and a basis for systems of classification; however, it contains less information than a description separately of the three responses.

The three responses of the original scale (developed in 1974), not the total score, should therefore be helpful in describing, monitoring and exchanging information about individual patients. Examination of the cranial nerves, in particular pupil reactivity, and neurological examination of the limbs, in particular the pattern and power of movement, provide supplementary information about the site and severity of localized brain damage.

The GCS and its derivative, the GCSS, are used widely for assessing patients, both before and after arrival at hospital. Extensive studies have supported their repeatability, validity and other clinimetric properties.

Traumatic brain injury

Traumatic brain injury (TBI) is the leading cause of death and disability around the globe and is therefore a major social, economic and health problem. It is the most frequent cause of coma and the leading cause of brain damage in children and young adults. In Europe it is responsible for more years of disability than any other cause.

Classification

- GCS of 13 or above is mild
- GCS of 9–12 is moderate
- GCS of 8 or below is severe (if no eye opening, this is called coma inducing)

Brain Trauma Foundation Guidelines: summary

Management guidelines emphasize admission of all 'salvageable' head injury patients to a specialist centre as this is associated with better outcomes. This association remains unexplained but could reflect the availability of specialized teams, including neurological intensive care. TBI patients require vigilance to prevent worsening of their neurological injury due to low blood pressure and hypoxaemia. Such events are called secondary physiological insults and are the focus of neurological critical care efforts before and during NCCU admission. Intracranial pressure monitoring should be considered in all patients at risk of developing brain swelling and/or haematoma development or expansion, the last two mandating neurosurgical review.

The outcomes from randomized controlled trials of titrated hypothermia (www.eurotherm3235trial.eu) and of decompressive craniectomy (rescue ICP) are eagerly awaited.

Subarachnoid haemorrhage (aneurysmal)

Subarachnoid haemorrhage (SAH) is a neurological catastrophe that exacts a high burden of untimely death and long-term disability and which can have a protracted and unpredictable course. It is fraught with risks of secondary neurological deterioration from rebleeding, cerebral oedema, hydrocephalus and delayed cerebral ischaemia (DIND: delayed ischaemic neurological deficits). In many cases, neurological risk is compounded by cardiac dysfunction, lung injury, systemic inflammatory responses and metabolic-endocrine imbalance. Because of these concurrent neurological and multisystem risks, the acute management of poor grade SAH patients falls squarely within the realm of neurological critical care.

Outcome after SAH may depend on hospital-related factors; for example, increased survival is noted in centres treating larger numbers of patients. The management of SAH is a multidisciplinary effort in which intensive care physicians have a prominent role. It is important to implement therapies for which there is robust evidence, to avoid damaging interventions and to formally investigate potential or current strategies that lack an adequate evidence base (Box 10.1).

Box 10.1 **Evidence-based subarachnoid haemorrhage management**

Beneficial interventions
Endovascular coiling when both coiling and clipping are suitable
Referral to a high volume centre
Early aneurysm repair
Use of nimodipine
Lung protective ventilation for acute lung injury

Ineffective and/or harmful interventions
Glucocorticoids
Antiepileptic drugs in all patients
Antifibrinolytic agents
Triple-H therapy to prevent vasospasm

Practices based on insufficient data
Use of CTA vs DSA to detect aneurysm
Blood pressure reduction to prevent aneurysm re-bleeding
Tight glycaemic control
Therapeutic hypothermia
Triple-H therapy to reverse vasospasm
Use of non-saline volume expanders
Blood transfusion triggers
Endovascular therapy as a first line in the treatment of vasospasm

Acute ischaemic stroke

Acute ischaemic stroke (AIS) causes considerable mortality and morbidity. There are over 1 million patients with acute new strokes each year in the European Union (EU). It is estimated that there will be 8.5 million patients with acute ischaemic stroke in the EU and USA over the next decade.

Prevention of secondary insults, including hypoxia and hypotension, is of great importance during periods of acute cerebral ischaemia in order to prevent worsening of the neurological injury. The most common causes of these are airway obstruction, hypoventilation, aspiration pneumonia and lung atelectasis. Patients with a decreased level of consciousness or brainstem stroke have an increased risk of airway compromise due to impaired oropharyngeal mobility and loss of protective reflexes.

Critical care has much to offer certain patients after AIS. However, for many interventions including thrombolysis and decompressive hemicraniectomy, the therapeutic time window is in the early phase after onset and this requires prompt recognition of the onset of the stroke and a healthcare system that facilitates early imaging with expert radiological interpretation. Even in advanced or well-funded healthcare systems, this standard is not consistently achieved.

Intracerebral haemorrhage

Non-traumatic intracerebral haemorrhage (ICH) is a major public health problem with an annual incidence of 10–30 per 100 000 population. Hospital admissions for ICH have increased by 18% in the past 10 years.

Observational studies show that about 30% of patients with supratentorial haemorrhage and almost all patients with brainstem or cerebellar haemorrhage have either decreased consciousness or bulbar muscle dysfunction necessitating endotracheal intubation. International guidelines are available for the management of hydration, nutrition, hyperglycaemia, hyperthermia, prevention of complications and early rehabilitation.

The volume of the ICH influences outcome. As a third of acute ICHs enlarge within 24 hours of onset; early treatment with a haemostatic drug may therefore improve outcomes. Phase II trials of recombinant Factor seven a (rFVIIa) were promising, but rFVIIa did not improve clinical outcome in a larger phase III trial with broader inclusion criteria. Systematic review has shown that evacuation of a spontaneous supratentorial intracerebral haemorrhage improves outcomes (odds ratio for death 0.71, 95% confidence interval 0.58–0.88).

Non-traumatic coma

Coma is one of the most common problems encountered in intensive care medicine and accounts for a substantial proportion of admissions. Coma, in the clinical sense, is defined as a deep sleep-like state from which the patient cannot be roused. Application of the general principles described above is mandatory while the aetiology is sought. Imaging is the cornerstone of investigation and is discussed later in the chapter.

Chemical–toxicological analysis of blood and urine, arterial blood gas analysis, electroencephalogram (EEG) and cerebrospinal fluid (CSF) examination are useful tools in the diagnosis of coma. Lumbar puncture is performed less frequently than in the past because neuroimaging can effectively exclude intracerebral and subarachnoid haemorrhages that are severe enough to cause coma (Box 10.2).

Box 10.2 Causes of non-traumatic coma

Structural
Non-traumatic intracranial haemorrhage
Ischaemic stroke
Venous thrombosis
Infection (abscess, subdural empyema, focal encephalitis)
Tumour (primary or metastatic)
Demyelination (acute demyelinating encephalomyelitis, multiple sclerosis)
Subarachnoid haemorrhage
Aneurysm in posterior fossa with mass effect
Pregnancy and puerperal problems (stroke, pituitary apoplexy, venous thrombosis, intracranial haemorrhage)

Diffuse
Hypoxic-ischaemic encephalopathy
Hypertensive encephalopathy (including eclampsia)
Pregnancy and puerperal problems (eclampsia, hypertensive encephalopathy, migraine, carbamoyltransferase deficiency carrier state)
Infection (meningitis, diffuse encephalitis)
Autoimmune disease (vasculitis)
Paraneoplastic syndromes (brain-stem and limbic encephalitis, vasculitis)
Toxic and metabolic (Box 10.1)
Seizure (post-ictal state, non-convulsive status epilepticus)
Others
Disordered temperature regulation (narcoleptic malignant syndrome, hypothermia)
Basilar migraine
High-altitude cerebral oedema (HACE)
Psychiatric (conversion, depression, mania, catatonia)

Infection (encephalitis, meningitis, abscess)

Meningitis

The most common symptoms of meningitis are headache and neck stiffness associated with fever, confusion or altered consciousness, vomiting, and an inability to tolerate light (photophobia) or loud noises (phonophobia). Sometimes, especially in small children, only non-specific symptoms may be present, such as irritability and drowsiness.

A lumbar puncture is used to diagnose or exclude meningitis (after a brain CT scan to assess risk of herniation). In immunocompromised patients, opportunistic infections should be considered: TB (including multidrug-resistant forms), HIV, cryptococcus, listeria, etc.

Empirical antibiotics must be started immediately, even before the results of the lumbar puncture and CSF analysis are known. The choice of initial treatment depends largely on the geographic region and local bacterial resistances. In the UK empirical treatment is with a third-generation cephalosporin such as cefotaxime or ceftriaxone. In the young and those over 50 years of age, as well as those who are immunocompromised, the addition of ampicillin or amoxicillin is recommended to cover *Listeria monocytogenes*. Encephalitis is treated by the addition of aciclovir. There are some data to support steroid administration where pneumococcal infection is suspected.

Seizure control

Emergency treatment of patients with status epilepticus involves monitoring respiratory and cardiovascular function closely and supporting as necessary. First-line treatment for patients with convulsive status epilepticus is an intravenous benzodiazepine (lorazepam or diazepam) followed by phenytoin. If this first-line therapy fails, patients should be referred to intensive care. An 'anaesthetic agent' is administered to abolish seizure activity, and this necessitates endotracheal intubation, mechanical ventilation and blood pressure stabilization. Seizures can be suppressed by infusion of an anaesthetic, commonly propofol and occasionally thiopental. Continuous EEG monitoring is desirable (Figure 10.1).

Muscle weakness

Failure of muscle power can lead to loss of airway protection and a requirement for mechanical ventilation. Careful consideration should be made to appropriateness of ICU admission in chronic degenerative diseases, but it should be noted that there is an increasing recognition of the utility of long-term ventilation in the community and the need for domiciliary ventilation services for patients with chronic neurological or neuromuscular disease resulting in ventilatory failure.

Guillain–Barré syndrome and myasthenia gravis are common causes of acquired weakness. The former presents additional challenges, including neuropathic pain control, autonomic disturbance, bowel and bladder dysfunction and the ever-present risk of infection and sepsis.

Imaging

In most causes of coma (once hypoglycaemia has been excluded) a CT scan of the brain is the first test performed after the physical examination. Intracranial haemorrhage, focal infection, tumour, hydrocephalus and various non-infectious inflammatory disorders may be identified by means of a CT scan of the brain with radiographic contrast. A magnetic resonance imaging sequence with gadolinium contrast will greatly increase the yield for abscesses, tumours, most non-infectious inflammatory lesions and demyelinating diseases. Magnetic resonance imaging may also increase the sensitivity for detecting brainstem lesions. Diffusion-weighted imaging can be very useful in the early determination of the presence and extent of ischaemic injury and when combined with perfusion-weighted imaging can reveal an imbalance in the two

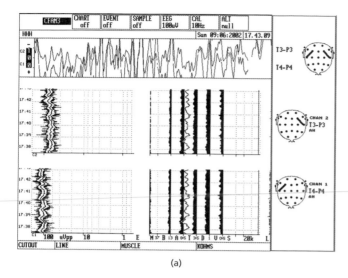

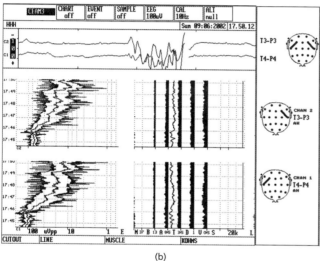

(a)

(b)

Figure 10.1 Processed electroencephalogram trace, time domain analysis, frequency analysis and amplitude (semi-logarithmic scale). (a) Status epilepticus; (b) after administration of an anaesthetic agent.

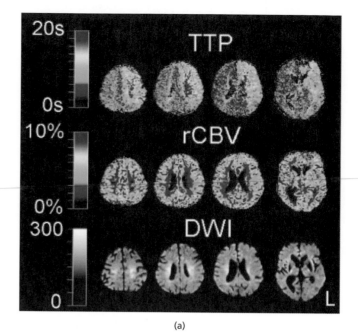

(a)

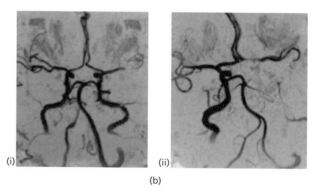

(i) (ii)

(b)

Figure 10.2 Patient with an acute right middle cerebral territory infarct, demonstrating a large ischaemic penumbra perfusion-weighted imaging (PWI) (perfusion lesion)> diffusion-weighted imaging (DWI) (diffusion lesion). The magnetic resonance angiogram (MRA) shows an occluded right middle cerebral artery.

deficits (DWI<PWI) that may represent penumbra tissue that is potentially salvageable (Figure 10.2). It may be complementary and helpful in making the decision of whether or not to administer thrombolysis to a patient.

Conclusion

In addition to managing critical illness of the nervous system, neurological critical care specialists also treat the medical complications that occur in such patients, including those affecting the heart, lungs, kidneys or any other organ systems, including treatment of infections. Most neurocritical care units are a collaborative effort between neurointensivists, neurosurgeons, neurologists, radiologists, pharmacists, physiotherapists and critical care nurses who all work together in order to provide coordinated care for the critically ill neurological patient.

Further reading

Andrews PJ, Citerio G, Longhi L, *et al.* Neuro-Intensive Care and Emergency Medicine (NICEM) Section of the European Society of Intensive Care Medicine. NICEM consensus on neurological monitoring in acute neurological disease. *Intensive Care Med.* 2008; 34:1362–70.

Elliott J, Smith M. The acute management of intracerebral hemorrhage: a clinical review. *Anesth Analg* 2010; 110:1419–27.

Sinclair HL, Andrews PJD. Bench-to-bedside review: hypothermia in traumatic brain injury. *Critical Care* 2010; 14:204. http://ccforum.com/14/1/204

Teasdale G, Jennett B. Assessment of coma and impaired consciousness. A practical scale. *Lancet* 1974; 2:81–4.

Young N, Rhodes JK, Mascia L, Andrews PJ. Ventilatory strategies for patients with acute brain injury. *Curr Opin Crit Care* 2010; 16:45–52.

https://www.braintrauma.org/pdf/protected/Guidelines_Management_2007w_bookmarks.pdf.

CHAPTER 11

Liver Support

Julia Wendon and Chris Holland

King's College Hospital, London, UK

> **OVERVIEW**
>
> - The mortality rate for acute liver failure ranges between 56% and 80%
> - The main role of intensive care is multi-organ support
> - The commonest cause of acute liver failure in the developed world is paracetamol (acetaminophen) toxicity
> - Hepatic encephalopathy is no longer the main cause of death but its detection and management require sophisticated cardiovascular and cerebral monitoring
> - Hepatorenal failure is due to the complex interplay between splanchnic, renal and systemic circulatory responses to liver failure. Terlipressin has been shown to be of use in its management
> - Novel hepatic replacement therapies are under development but definitive studies as to their efficacy are, as yet, unpublished

Introduction

Liver failure is a relatively rare but devastating cause of critical illness, its definitive treatment remains orthotopic liver transplantation (OLT). There is an international shortage of donor organs and this directs intensive care practice towards largely supportive care and acting as a bridge to transplant. Nearly every body system suffers either directly or indirectly from hepatic disease and such patients frequently require multi-system support. Despite strenuous efforts, mortality statistics range from 56% to over 80% in centres where transplantation is not possible.

Classification and aetiology

A temporal classification of acute liver failure has been described: hyperacute, 7 days; acute, 7–28 days; and subacute, 28 days to 6 months. Chronic liver disease can progress to end-stage disease insidiously or with an acute-on-chronic time-scale. One time-scale suggested for defining acute-on-chronic liver failure has been 2–4 weeks, obviously leaving much room for overlap. The rate of evolution does not usually suggest the likely cause or prognosis. Over the past half century the spectrum of liver failure precipitants has changed (Figure 11.1) so that the leading cause of hyperacute liver failure in the developed world is now acute paracetamol (acetaminophen) toxicity. This carries a relatively good prognosis given appropriate therapy. In the developing world infection with one of the hepatitis viruses still remains the predominant cause.

> Box 11.1 **Model of end-stage liver disease (MELD)**
>
> $3.8 \times \log_e [\text{bilirubin (mg/dL)}] + 11.2 \times \log_e(\text{INR}) + 9.6 \times \log_e [\text{creatinine (mg/dL)}] + 6.4 \times \text{aetiology}^*$
>
> *Aetiology: 0 if cholestatic or alcoholic, 1 otherwise
> Online worksheet available at www.mayo.edu/int-med/gi/model/mayomodl.htm

---

There are several measures of the severity of liver failure. The model of end-stage liver disease (MELD) (Box 11.1) attempts to prognosticate end-stage chronic disease. The Glasgow Alcohol Hepatitis Score (Table 11.1) is condition specific whereas the King's College Liver Transplant Criteria (Table 11.2) uses historical data to assess the urgency of transplant. These, and other, scoring systems continue to be refined and validated. Systems that use objective markers of multi-system dysfunction appear more accurate at predicting outcome than those which use subjective measures or solely hepatic markers.

Diagnosis

Formal diagnosis of acute liver failure is made by an increase in the prothrombin time (PT) of 4–6 seconds (international

Table 11.1 The Glasgow alcoholic hepatitis score.

	Score given		
	1	**2**	**3**
Age	<50	≥ 50	–
White cell count (10⁹/L)	<15	≥ 15	–
Urea (mmol/L)	<5	5	–
PT ratio	<1.5	1.5–2.0	>2.0
Bilirubin (micromol/L)	<125	125–250	>250

PT, prothrombin time.

ABC of Intensive Care, Second Edition.
Edited by Graham R. Nimmo and Mervyn Singer.
© 2011 Blackwell Publishing Ltd. Published 2011 by Blackwell Publishing Ltd.

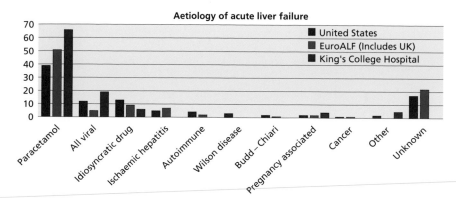

Figure 11.1 Aetiologies of liver failure in the developed world.

Table 11.2 King's College criteria.

Paracetamol-induced acute liver failure	Non-paracetamol aetiology
pH <7.3 following volume resuscitation irrespective of grade of encephalopathy	PT >100 s (INR >6.5)
Or	
Concurrent findings of:	Any three of the following:
Grade III-IV encephalopathy	Aetiology: seronegative hepatitis or drug-induced liver failure
Creatinine >300 µmol/L	Age <10 or >40 years
PT >100 s (INR >6.5)	Jaundice to encephalopathy >7 days
Serum lactate >3.5 mmol/L at 4 h or >3 mmol/L at 12 h	Bilirubin >300 µmol/L PT >50 s (INR >3.5)

PT, prothrombin time.

normalization ratio (INR) >1.5) and the development of hepatic encephalopathy (HE). Once the diagnosis is made, a careful search for possible aetiologies is necessary. A corroborating history may be difficult to obtain in the presence of HE. The spectrum of aetiologies is reflected in the battery of suggested initial investigations (Box 11.2).

> **Box 11.2 Suggested initial laboratory analysis**
>
> Initial laboratory analysis
>
> - Prothrombin time/INR
> - Blood chemistry
> - Sodium, potassium, chloride, bicarbonate, calcium, magnesium, phosphate, glucose
> - AST, ALT, alkaline phosphatase, gamma GT, total bilirubin, albumin, creatinine, urea
> - Arterial blood gas
> - Arterial lactate
> - Full blood count
> - Blood type and screen
> - Paracetamol (acetaminophen) level
> - Toxicology screen
> - Viral hepatitis serologies

> - Anti-HAV IgM, HBSAg, anti-HBc IgM, anti-HEV, anti-HCV
> - Ceruloplasmin level
> - Pregnancy test
> - Ammonia (arterial if possible)
> - Autoimmune markers
> - Anti-nuclear antibodies, Anti-smooth muscle antibodies, immunoglobulin levels
> - HIV status
> - Amylase and lipase

Several precipitants of acute liver failure have specific antidotes or suggested therapies that will improve prognosis if initiated promptly (Table 11.3).

Coagulopathy

The coagulopathy of liver disease arises not only because of the failure to produce clotting factors II, V, VII and IX but also because of the failure of the diseased liver to clear activated clotting factors. In chronic liver disease a degree of hypersplenism and thrombocytopenia often adds to the coagulopathy, especially if disseminated intravascular coagulation (DIC) co-exists. The degree of coagulopathy is a measure of the severity of liver disease and of patient prognosis. Correction of coaguloapthy is therefore not routinely indicated unless necessitated by active bleeding or planned interventions. Careful selection of appropriate means of correction can reduce the total volume transfused and allow continued use of the INR as a monitor of patient progress.

Table 11.3 Recommended specific antidotes.

Aetiology	Therapy
Paracetamol (acetaminophen)	Intravenous *N*-acetyl cysteine
Hepatitis B	Lamivudine/adefovir
Autoimmune	Immunosuppression
Budd–Chiari syndrome	Anticoagulation Transjugular intrahepatic portosystemic shunt
Amanita phalloides	Penicillin/silymarin

Hepatic encephalopathy

HE remains incompletely understood. Four compatible theories have been suggested: cerebral oedema secondary to cerebral vasomotor dysfunction, oedema secondary to ammonia toxicity, inflammation due to systemic inflammatory response syndrome (SIRS) and the accumulation of putative benzodiazepine-like molecules. HE is graded on a scale of I to IV (Table 11.4). Distinguishing between the various grades of encephalopathy requires careful patient assessment using easily replicated tools.

Deterioration in HE grade can occur suddenly and may indicate the presentation of a disastrous intracranial pathology. Patients with grade II HE should be managed in a high dependency environment. Grades III and IV HE requires definitive airway protection and appropriate monitoring. Grade IV HE is strongly associated with elevated levels of serum ammonia, a high incidence of raised intracranial pressure and the development of uncal herniation. Management aims should be to maintain adequate cerebral oxygenation without inducing intracranial hyperaemia. General tenets of neuroprotective care therefore apply (Table 11.5). Institution of active management of cerebral metabolic demand, oxygen supply and perfusion pressure may require specialized methods of monitoring these parameters.

Table 11.4 Grade of encephalopathy, corresponding clinical features and approximate Glasgow Coma Score (GCS).

Encephalopathy grade	Clinical features	GCS
0	Normal	15
I	Shortened attention span Minimal lack of awareness	15–14
II	Minimal temporo-spatial disorientation Inappropriate behaviour	13–11
III	Overt confusion Gross disorientation Somnolence but responsive to verbal stimuli	10–8
IV	Unresponsive to verbal stimuli Pupillary abnormalities	< 83

Table 11.5 Targets and strategies for cerebral protection.

Target	Strategy
Cerebral perfusion pressure	Cerebral blood flow Fluid resuscitation Vasopressor agents Osmodiuretics and electrolyte balance Normocapnia Head-up bed tilt/avoidance of neck ligatures
Normoxia	Ventilation and transfusion
Reduction in cerebral metabolism	Anaesthetic agents Antiepileptic agents Avoidance of fever – ?Hypothermia
Uncertain mechanism	Normoglycaemia Magnesium therapy

Seizure activity, both clinical and subclinical, may occur. Seizures should be controlled promptly as they increase cerebral oxygen demand and intracranial pressure. Seizure control with benzodiazepines will result in sedation, making it difficult to monitor the progression of HE. Phenytoin has been recommended as the agent of choice for seizure control in these circumstances. Prophylactic phenytoin has not proven to be of any benefit. With intensive, multisystem support HE has ceased to be the main cause of death from acute liver failure over the past two decades.

Another method of controlling cerebral metabolic disarray may be induced hypothermia. Hypothermia below 32–33°C has been used in other pathologies to achieve a degree of neuroprotection. However, when studied in critically ill patients with liver disease, it is associated with an unacceptably high degree of cardiovascular instability and a worsening of coagulopathy. Studies are ongoing regarding the safety and efficacy of more moderate hypothermia of 33–34°C.

Cardiovascular management

Many patients with liver failure present with, or even because of, haemodynamic instability. The direct cardiovascular sequelae of liver failure tend to result in a high cardiac output, low systemic vascular resistance and a relatively hypovolaemic picture. In acute liver dysfunction, patients with surviving renal function may become hypernatraemic due to the resulting water and salt retention. Adequate resuscitation with crystalloid and colloid fluids and vasopressor support as required needs invasive monitoring. Requirement for vasopressor support may be modified by administration of replacement doses of hydrocortisone. Formal testing for cortisol deficiency is sometimes used in this situation.

Renal dysfunction

Often the clinical picture is worsened by renal dysfunction, either due to direct renal injury or the hepato-renal syndrome (HRS). HRS is categorized into two types according to the speed of onset. Type 1 HRS has an acute evolution and is associated with a worse prognosis. HRS may be due to splanchnic vasodilatation worsening renal perfusion in the presence of intense extra-hepatic vasoconstriction. Systemic vasoconstriction is driven by the renin angiotensin and sympathetic nervous systems in response to the cardiovascular picture described above. The splanchnic vasodilatation may be due to increased endotoxin, complement and nitric oxide levels within the portal circulation. In patients with pre-existing cirrhosis this vasomotor and neuroendocrine response results in hyponatraemia, rather than the hypernatraemia often seen in acutely unwell patients. Renal dysfunction and failure should be treated with appropriate fluid resuscitation and the initiation of renal replacement therapy. Continuous haemofiltration, rather than intermittent dialysis, is often better tolerated in haemodynamically unstable patients. Vasoconstrictor therapy with alpha-adrenergic agonists or vasopressin has been shown to ameliorate or even reverse the evolution of HRS. More recently, terlipressin, a vasopressin analogue, has been shown to be efficacious in treating renal, systemic, portal and possibly intracranial vascular dysfunction

Sepsis

Infection may be the initiating event of liver failure while intercurrent sepsis is also a common problem. Impaired immune function, in part secondary to reduced complement factor production and impaired neutrophil, leucocyte and monocyte function, can result in a delayed presentation of the clinical signs of infection. The interventions required for diagnosis and management of liver disease also increase patient vulnerability to invasive infection. Choice of antibiotic should be guided by local microbiological surveillance. The high incidence of mycoses in patients with liver dysfunction should prompt a low threshold for the use of antifungal agents.

Only patients who have an episode of gastrointestinal bleeding or an episode of spontaneous bacterial peritonitis (SBP) have been shown to have a significant outcome benefit from prophylactic antibiotics. Concerns regarding the evolution of resistance with long-term exposure to antimicrobials therefore justify a more pragmatic policy of having a low-threshold for commencing time-limited courses of broad-spectrum antibiotics. Microbiological investigation should then be used to narrow the spectrum wherever possible.

Gastrointestinal and metabolic management

Patients with both acute and chronic liver disease are at increased risk of gastrointestinal (GI) bleeding. Ventilation for more than 48 hours, coagulopathy, sepsis and shock are all associated with this complication. In addition, the formation of porto-systemic shunts is associated with variceal bleeding. The incidence of GI bleeding and ventilator-associated pneumonia are reduced with pharmacological gastric protection, although acid reduction therapy may be associated with an increased rate of *Clostridium difficile* infection.

Gastric protection may also be afforded by the institution of enteral feeding. This route of calorie delivery to patients who are often catabolic and critically ill is also preferred to the parenteral route in many centres for reasons related to infection, fluid balance and the tendency for parenteral nutrition to provide excessive caloric amounts. Glycaemic control is often poor in patients with liver dysfunction. This may be secondary to reduced glycogen stores, decreased gluconeogenesis and high levels of endogenous insulin. For this reason continuous intravenous glucose infusion is often used, at least until continuous enteral feeding is established. Tight glycaemic control has not been proven to be of benefit in patients with critical liver disease; however, hyperglycaemia worsens neurological outcomes and should be avoided. Other nutritional considerations should include adequate provision of vitamins, minerals and trace elements.

The avoidance of constipation is important as it increases the risk of bacterial translocation, increased portal and sinusoidal pressures and the risk of GI haemorrhage and sepsis. Non-absorbable disaccharides are often used, particularly if patients have HE. It was postulated that the mode of action of these agents would, in addition, promote the enteric excretion of ammonia and prevent its absorption from the gut. A recent literature review has suggested that non-absorbable disaccharides may not offer any additional benefit compared with other aperients.

Phosphate, magnesium, calcium and potassium levels are frequently low in patients who are critically ill with liver disease. This can be worsened in the context of large fluid losses and renal replacement therapy. Electrolyte imbalances should be actively sought and corrected. Recently, serum phosphate levels have attracted some attention. Hypophosphataemia is commonly seen in acute liver failure. The mechanism of its development is unclear but may relate to increased renal loss, abnormal distribution or increased consumption by a metabolically active, regenerating liver. Hyperphosphataemia in acute hepatic paracetamol (acetaminophen) toxicity seems to be associated with a worse outcome.

Liver support devices

Given the poor prognosis and potential for disastrous deterioration that might make a patient untransplantable while waiting for a transplant organ, much interest has focused on the potential for artificial liver assist or replacement technologies. Currently, two approaches exist: wholly artificial devices that attempt to replicate the detoxification activities of the liver, and devices that incorporate hepatocytes of human or other species of origin that attempt to also replicate the liver's synthetic and metabolic functions. These devices remain experimental and large-scale Phase two and three trials are awaited.

Emergency surgery

In patients with acute liver failure few emergency surgical interventions are indicated other than OLT or for specific indications. In the acutely unwell patient with pre-existing cirrhosis, emergency decompression of the portal vasculature may offer some benefit, but carries with it the increased risks of surgery in the critically ill patient and possible worsening of hepatic encephalopathy.

Conclusion

Patients with acute liver failure have a poor prognosis. Their condition requires multisystem support, complex treatments and monitoring. Transplantation often represents the best hope of a definitive treatment but is not usually immediately available. The commonest cause of acute liver failure in the developed world is now paracetamol (acetaminophen) toxicity. With expert care, an increasing number of patients are now supported giving time for their native liver to regenerate.

Further reading

Bernal W, Auzinger G, Sizer E, Wendon J. Intensive care management of acute liver failure. *Semin Liver Dis* 2008; 28:188–200.

Canabal JM, Kramer DJ. Management of sepsis in patients with liver failure. *Curr Opin Crit Care* 2008; 14:189–97.

Polson J, Lee WM. AASLD position paper: the management of acute liver failure. *Hepatology* 2005; 41:1179–97.

Ruiz-del-Arbol L, Monescillo A, Arocena C, *et al.* Circulatory function and hepatorenal syndrome in cirrhosis. *Hepatology* 2005; 42:439–47.

Shawcross D, Jalan R. Dispelling myths in the treatment of hepatic encephalopathy. *Lancet* 2005; 365:431–3.

Online tutorial

There is an online tutorial on this subject at http://www.scottish intensivecare.org.uk/education/index.htm. Click on the 'Induction tutorials' tab to find it.

CHAPTER 12

Gastrointestinal Support

Saif Al Musa and Tony M. Rahman

St George's Hospital, London, UK

OVERVIEW

- Gastrointestinal motility is frequently disturbed throughout the gut from oesophagus to colon, resulting in reflux, diarrhoea, ileus and a failure to meet nutritional goals
- Gastrointestinal haemorrhage commonly occurs as a result of stress-related mucosal damage
- Prophylactic measures and early recognition help reduce the impact of gastrointestinal complications

---

Box 12.1 **Risk factors associated with gastrointestinal bleeds on ICU**

- Respiratory failure and mechanical ventilation> 48 h
- Coagulopathy/thrombocytopenia
- Haemodynamic compromise/hypotension
- Severe hepatic disease
- Severe renal disease
- Major trauma/burns
- Multiple organ dysfunction

Introduction

Gastrointestinal dysfunction in the critically ill is common and occurs as a result of interactions between the underlying illness, sepsis, organ failure and treatments initiated to support the unwell patient. Compromise of gastrointestinal blood flow and oxygen delivery is important, leading to serious complications including haemorrhage, ischaemia, dysmotility and multiple organ dysfunction syndrome (MODS). The clinical assessment of gastrointestinal complications in the critically ill is shown in Table 12.1.

Upper gastrointestinal bleeding

Gastrointestinal bleeds mostly occur in the upper gastrointestinal tract and are associated with significant morbidity and mortality. Causes of upper gastrointestinal bleeds are listed in Table 12.2. The presentation of variceal/ulcer bleeds may be asymptomatic, occult, overt or life threatening and several risk factors have been identified (Box 12.1). Clinically relevant bleeds occur in up to 0.7% of critically ill patients with most occurring during the first 2 weeks following ICU admission. Following a non-variceal bleed, various validated scoring systems, for example Rockall, Blatchford and Baylor, can be used to predict outcome (Table 12.3).

The commonest cause, stress-related mucosal damage (SRMD), results in overt bleeding in 25% of patients not receiving acid suppression. SRMD typically affects the fundal region and is evident in more than 70% of patients within 24 hours of ICU admission. Currently, ranitidine is the drug of choice for stress ulcer prophylaxis; however, the use of proton pump inhibitors is on the increase. Concerns have been expressed at the association between acid suppression medication and ventilator-acquired pneumonia (VAP) and *Clostridium difficile* (*C. difficile*) infection.

The investigation of upper gastrointestinal bleeding involves fibreoptic endoscopy. In those instances in which no cause is found a colonoscopy and/or mesenteric angiogram and/or labelled red cell scan may be required. During endoscopy several therapeutic options are available dependent on the haemorrhagic site (Table 12.4). In addition, mesenteric angiography and embolization may be used to arrest severe haemorrhage from the bowel. This technique may be used when endoscopic investigations have not localized a source of bleeding, or when endoscopic techniques have failed, when the bleeding site is inaccessible to endoscopic therapies, or pre-emptively to avoid surgery (Table 12.4).

Intravenous proton pump inhibitors are advocated in patients with ulcers that have stigmata of recent haemorrhage. They have been shown to reduce the risk of rebleeding and the need for repeat endoscopy and/or surgery. *Helicobacter pylori* (*H. pylori*) eradication therapy may also be required. Currently, this is administered empirically to patients with duodenal ulcers. However its use in gastric ulcers is restricted to those with evidence of infection. Post-gastrointestinal bleed, *H. pylori* can be detected by several methods, including serology, histology and stool antigen testing. The last technique has been shown to have utility in the critically ill patient.

ABC of Intensive Care, Second Edition.
Edited by Graham R. Nimmo and Mervyn Singer.
© 2011 Blackwell Publishing Ltd. Published 2011 by Blackwell Publishing Ltd.

Table 12.1 Clinical assessment for gastrointestinal complications.

Assessment of ICU patient	Gastrointestinal association/complication
General	
Admitting diagnosis e.g. head injury	Delayed gastric emptying
Heart rate/rhythm e.g. atrial fibrillation	Mesenteric ischaemia
Blood pressure-hypotension	Haemorrhage/ischaemia
Mechanical ventilation settings/duration	Haemorrhage/ischaemia
Supine position	Gastro-oesophageal reflux
Elevated capillary blood glucose	Delayed gastric emptying
Gastrointestinal	
Oral cavity	Dental hygiene/peri-oral injury from tracheal tube
Tube feeding (nasogastric/nasojejunal)	Gastro-oesophageal reflux Diarrhoea
Nasogastric aspirates	Delayed gastric emptying
Increasing abdominal distension	Small/large bowel ileus Intra-abdominal hypertension
Bruising in loins and umbilicus	Pancreatitis
Tenderness	Ileus/ischaemia/peritonitis
Bowel sounds:	
Increased	Ileus
Absent	Peritonitis
Bowel output	Constipation/diarrhoea/malaena/ fresh blood
Drugs	
Stress ulcer prophylaxis	Diarrhoea
Antibiotics	Diarrhoea
Inotropes (dopamine/adrenaline)	Delayed gastric emptying Diarrhoea
Opioids	Delayed gastric emptying Constipation

Table 12.2 Causes of upper gastrointestinal bleeds on ICU (%).

Stress-related mucosal damage/gastric and duodenal ulcers/gastritis/duodenitis	38
Oesophageal varices	26
Not identified	16
Oesophagitis	14
Mallory Weiss	2
Haemobilia	1
Others (including angiodysplasia, malignancy)	4

Variceal bleeds normally occur in patients with advanced liver disease and are associated with high mortality rates (up to 50%). Varices develop as a result of portal hypertension. On presentation, patients may be taking, or can be commenced on, propanolol, which acts by reducing portal pressure. Hepatic venous wedge pressures of less than 12 mmHg are not normally associated with variceal haemorrhage.

In the event of an acute variceal bleed the potent vasoconstrictor terlipressin is used in conjunction with an endoscopic examination of the upper gastrointestinal tract. In those cases where therapeutic measures (banding and/or sclerotherapy) have been unsuccessful,

a Sengstaken–Blackmore tube or equivalent (e.g. Linton tube) and/or emergency surgery may be required. In addition to the initial treatment of variceal bleeds, prophylactic antibiotics are required to reduce the risk of sepsis.

Lower gastrointestinal haemorrhage

Lower gastrointestinal bleeds are less common and predominantly affect the left side of the colon. Causes of lower gastrointestinal bleeds are shown in Box 12.2. Diagnosis can be made using computed tomography, angiography and/or colonoscopy. Most causes (>80%) stop spontaneously. However, in some instances, embolization, endoscopic ablation and/or surgery may be required.

Box 12.2 **Causes of lower gastrointestinal bleeds on ICU**

- Infective colitis
- Inflammatory bowel disease
- Ischaemic colitis
- Acute haemorrhagic rectal ulcers
- Pseudomembranous colitis
- Diverticular disease
- Angiodysplasia
- Colorectal cancer/polyps
- Small bowel lesions
- Upper gastrointestinal bleeds

Normal gastrointestinal motility

Under normal physiological conditions the motility of the gut is divided into two patterns: fasting (interdigestive) and fed (digestive). The fasting pattern is characterized by the three phases of the migratory motor complex (MMC) that clears the stomach and small bowel of undigested food and bacteria. This function is disturbed in the critically ill and predisposes to reflux, diarrhoea, ileus and a failure to meet nutritional goals.

Gastro-oesophageal reflux

Gastro-oesophageal reflux (GOR) is commonly recognized in the critically ill patient and may exacerbate oesophagitis and VAP. Under normal conditions GOR is prevented by the actions of saliva, oesophageal motility and lower oesophageal sphincter tone, all of which may be disturbed in the critically ill (Box 12.3). Preventative measures that aim to reduce the impact of risk factors include the semi-recumbent position (45° angle) and the use of prokinetics.

Box 12.3 **Risk factors associated with gastro-oesophageal reflux**

- Reduced salivary flow
- Impaired oesophageal motility
- Reduced/absent lower oesophageal sphincter tone
- Impaired gastric emptying
- Bile reflux
- Nasogastric tubes
- Supine body position

Table 12.3 Rockall scoring system for upper gastrointestinal bleeds.

Parameters	Range of scores	Predicted outcome		
		Total score	Rebleed (%)	Mortality (%)
Age (range <60 to >80 years)	0–2			
Haemodynamic compromise (heart rate, blood pressure)	0–2	0–2	5	0
Pre-existing conditions (none – metastatic disease)	0–3	3–7	11–44	3–27
Endoscopic diagnosis (none – upper gastrointestinal malignancy)	0–2	>8	42	41
Endoscopic evidence of recent bleed (none – active bleeding)	0–2			

Table 12.4 Treatment options available for upper gastrointestinal bleeds.

Type of haemorrhage	Site of haemorrhage	Endoscopic treatments	Medical	Radiological
Variceal	Oesophageal	Banding Sclerotherapy	Intravenous terlipressin Recombinant Factor VIIa	Transjugular intrahepatic portosystemic shunts (TIPS)
	Gastric	Sclerotherapy		
Ulcer	Oesophageal Gastric Duodenal	Sclerotherapy (adrenaline) +/− Heater probe (diathermy) +/− Endoscopic clips	Intravenous/high dose oral Proton pump inhibitors/*Helicobacter pylori* eradication	Angiographic embolization
Angiodysplasia	Gastric	Heater probe (diathermy) Argon photocoagulation		

Gastroparesis

Clinically, gastroparesis is detected by gastric aspirates/gastric residual volumes (GRVs) of 150–500 mL after 4 hours of feeding. Treatment is directed at promoting gastric motility using prokinetics, metoclopramide, erythromycin or domperidone. In some instances, nasojejunal feeding may be required (Figure 12.1; Box 12.4).

Box 12.4 Risk factors associated with reduced gastric motility

- Admitting diagnosis, e.g. head injury, burns, trauma
- Advanced age
- Malnourished state
- Hyperglycaemia
- Impaired renal function
- Type of mechanical ventilation
- Opioids/inotropes use

Diarrhoea and constipation

Although the definition of diarrhoea in the critically ill has not been standardized, it is a common problem and has multiple causes, including enteral feed, malnutrition, hypoalbuminaemia, infections (e.g. *C. difficile*) and iatrogenic/drug induced (e.g. antacids, antibiotics, laxatives). Diarrhoea can result in a failure to meet nutritional goals, and can cause wound contamination and electrolyte imbalances. Supportive care may require intravenous fluid/electrolyte replacement therapy with or without oral rehydration salts. Practical management may entail the use of a rectal tube or other similar bowel management systems (Figure 12.2). Optimal treatment is directed towards the underlying cause.

The critically ill patient may also become constipated for several reasons, including post-surgery (ileus), sedatives, analgesia (especially opioids), immobility and dehydration. Treatment options include nasogastric tubes, rehydration, minimizing opioid use, stool softeners/enemas and flatus tubes.

Other important gastrointestinal conditions

Mesenteric ischaemia occurs in response to a disruption in the arterial blood supply to the gut from either non-obstructing (e.g. hypotension) or obstructing (e.g. embolus or thrombus) causes. Mesenteric ischaemia can result in lower gastrointestinal haemorrhage and peritonitis. Treatment requires fluid resuscitation, antibiotics and, often, laparotomy with definitive surgical intervention.

C. difficile infection is increasing in prevalence and severity, resulting in more patients requiring ICU admission either with or for this condition. The use of multiple antibiotics, acid suppressants and enteral feeds predispose patients to *C. difficile* infection. Diagnosis is made by the detection of toxins from stool samples or, more recently, polymerase chain reaction assays. Complications include lower gastrointestinal bleeds, ileus and megacolon (Figure 12.3). Treatment requires fluid replacement, barrier

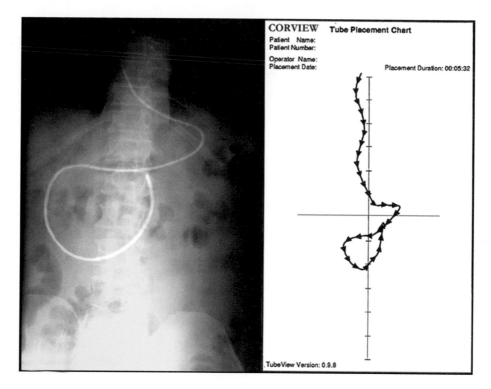

Figure 12.1 'Cortrak' nasojejunal feeding tube. Reproduced with permission from Viasys MedSystems, USA.

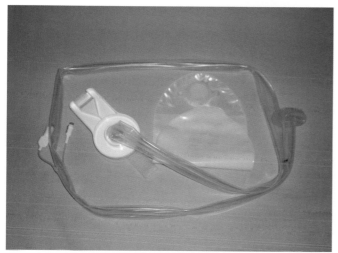

Figure 12.2 An example of a rectal tube.

Box 12.5 **Causes of acute pancreatitis**

- Gallstones
- Alcohol
- Traumatic injury
- Post surgery
- Drugs, e.g. azathioprine, steroids, tetracyclines, valproate
- Infections, e.g. viral hepatitis, mumps, Epstein–Barr virus
- Hypertriglyceridaemia
- Idiopathic

Treatment is supportive, and comprises fluids, analgesia, control of hyperglycaemia, nutritional support and stress ulcer prophylaxis.

nursing, isolation, enteral antibiotics and, if possible, rationalizing systemic antibiotic therapy. In severe cases surgery may be required.

Acute pancreatitis has several aetiologies (Box 12.5). Six per cent of patients admitted to hospital with this condition may require ICU admission. Those patients invariably have the severest forms of the disease, namely severe necrotizing or haemorrhagic pancreatitis. Diagnosis is based on clinical, biochemical and radiological findings (Table 12.5). The severity and predicted outcome can be assessed by several scoring systems including Ranson (Table 12.6), Imrie, Glasgow and APACHE II/III scores. A newer scoring system, the pancreatitis outcome prediction (POP) score, has recently been developed in the UK but requires further validation (Table 12.7).

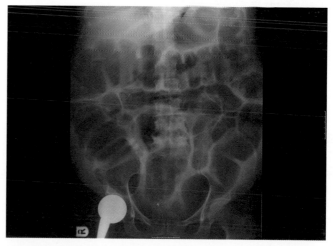

Figure 12.3 Abdominal radiograph of toxic megacolon secondary to *Clostridium difficile*.

Table 12.5 Diagnosis of acute pancreatitis.

Clinical	Epigastric pain radiating to back, nausea, vomiting
	Pyrexia, hypotension, tachycardia, abdominal guarding/tenderness, Grey–Turner's/Cullen's sign, reduced bowel sounds
Biochemical	Raised serum amylase (>3× upper limit of normal)
	Raised serum lipase (>3× upper limit of normal)
	Elevated urea
	Elevated hepatic transaminases
	Elevated blood glucose, elevated C-reactive protein
Radiological	Abdominal radiograph – Sentinel loop (rare)
	Ultrasound scan – help to identify cause, e.g. gallstones
	Computed tomography–severity graded A–E necrosis graded 0–6

Table 12.6 Ranson's scoring criteria for acute pancreatitis and predicted mortality.

Parameters on admission (one point/criteria)	Parameters after 48 h (one point/criteria)	Predicted mortality rate
Age in years >55 years	>10% fall in haematocrit	Score 0–2: 2%
		Score 3–4: 15%
		Score 5–6: 40%
		Score >7: 100%
White blood cell count >16 000/mm^3	Rise in blood urea nitrogen by >1.8 mmol/L (after IV fluid hydration)	
Blood glucose >11 mmol/L		
Serum aspartate transaminase >250 IU/L	Serum calcium <2.0 mmol/L	
Serum lactate dehydrogenase >350 IU/L	Arterial PO$_2$ <60 mmHg (<8.0 kPa)	
	Base deficit >4 mmol/L	
	Estimated fluid sequestration >6 L	

Table 12.7 Pancreatitis outcome prediction scoring criteria for severe acute pancreatitis and mortality.

Parameters during first 24 h	Range of scores	Predicted mortality rate
Age (range 16–>70)	0–8	
Mean arterial pressure (mmHg) (range <40–>90)	0–8	Total score 0–10: <20%
		Total score >20: >40%
		Total score >30: >80%
PiO$_2$/FiO$_2$ ratio (kPa) (range <10–>30)	0–4	
Arterial pH (range <7.0–>7.35)	0–10	
Serum urea (mmol/L) (range <5–>17)	0–6	
Total calcium (mmol/L) (range <1.6–>2.5)	0–4	

Table 12.8 Definitions associated with intra-abdominal pressure (IAP).

Normal intra-abdominal pressure	5–7 mmHg
Intra-abdominal hypertension (IAH)	Sustained/repeated IAP >12 mmHg
Abdominal compartment syndrome	IAH >20 mmHg + new onset organ failure
Severity of intra-abdominal hypertension	
Grade 1	12–15 mmHg
Grade 2	16–20 mmHg
Grade 3	21–25 mmHg
Grade 4	>25 mmHg

Early enteral feeding via the nasojejunal route is recommended for severe pancreatitis and is associated with reduced surgical intervention, mortality and more rapid restoration of gut motility. In those circumstances where enteral feeding is not feasible, total parenteral nutrition (perhaps with added glutamine) is required. The role and choice of prophylactic antibiotics remains controversial; while beta-lactams may confer some benefit, meta-analyses are inconsistent with respect to reducing rates of pancreatic necrosis and/or mortality. In some cases, radiologically guided drainage of pseudocysts and/or surgical debridement of the pancreas is required.

Acalculous cholecystitis occurs in up to 3% of patients and is associated with a high morbidity and mortality. Risk factors include shock, sepsis and prolonged mechanical ventilation. The diagnosis requires ultrasound and/or computed tomography scans. Treatment involves percutaneous drainage of the gall bladder.

Intra-abdominal hypertension occurs in approximately one-third of patients. Intra-abdominal pressure is measured via the bladder with values below 5–7 mmHg being regarded as normal (Table 12.8). Elevation of intra-abdominal pressure has profound metabolic and physiological effects that may lead to hypotension (reduced venous return), respiratory failure, oligo-anuric renal impairment and mesenteric ischaemia. Initially recognized in the setting of abdominal trauma, it has now been associated with surgical and medical complications in multi-organ failure. Causes of raised intra-abdominal pressure are listed in Box 12.6. Decompressive laparotomy may be required to treat it.

Box 12.6 **Causes of intra-abdominal hypertension**

- Trauma
- Intra-abdominal bleeding
- Ileus
- Acute pancreatitis
- Mesenteric ischaemia
- Massive fluid replacement
- Use of inotropes

In summary, disturbances in normal gut function are associated with important clinical consequences in the critically ill. Gastrointestinal complications commonly occur in this cohort resulting in significant morbidity and mortality. The spectrum of disease is vast and can affect any part of the gut. Early detection and recognition of the appropriate clinical features together with the correct investigation/treatment is required to help reduce and manage the burden of gastrointestinal disorders in the critically ill.

Further reading

Chapman MJ, Nguyen NQ, Fraser RJL. Gastrointestinal motility and prokinetics in the critically ill. *Curr Opin Crit Care* 2007; 13:187–94.

Harrison DA, D'Amico G, Singer M. The Pancreatitis Outcome Prediction (POP) Score: a new prognostic index for patients with severe acute pancreatitis. *Crit Care Med* 2007; 35:1703–8.

Lin CC, Lee YC, Lee H, *et al.* Bedside colonoscopy for critically ill patients with acute lower gastrointestinal bleeding. *Intensive Care Med* 2005; 31:743–6.

Liu TH, Kwong KL, Tamm, EP, *et al.* Acute pancreatitis in intensive care unit patients: value of clinical and radiologic prognosticators at predicting clinical course and outcome *Crit Care Med* 2003; 31:1026–30.

Martin B. Prevention of gastrointestinal complications in the critically ill patient. *AACN Adv Crit Care* 2007; 18:158–66.

Maury E, Tankovic J, Ebel A, Offenstadt G; Parisian Group of the Upper Gastrointestinal Bleeding Survey. An observational study of upper gastrointestinal bleeding in intensive care units: is *Helicobacter pylori* the culprit? *Crit Care Med.* 2005; 33:1513–8.

Mutlu GM, Mutlu EA, Factor P. GI complications in patients receiving mechanical ventilation. *Chest* 2001; 119:1222–41.

Plaiser PW, Van Buuren HR, Bruining HA. Upper gastrointestinal endoscopy at four intensive care units in one hospital: frequency and indication. *Eur J Gastroenterol Hepatol* 1998; 10:997–1000.

Rockall TA, Logan RF, Devlin HB, Northfield TC. Risk assessment after acute upper gastrointestinal haemorrhage. *Gut* 1996; 38:316–21.

CHAPTER 13

Nutrition in the ICU

Marcia McDougall

Queen Margaret Hospital, Dunfermline, UK

OVERVIEW

- To understand the importance of feeding in the critically ill
- To understand the practical issues involved in prescribing and delivering feed

Nutritional goals and challenges in the critically ill

The goals of nutritional support are detection of pre-existing malnutrition, prevention of deficiency-related morbidity and further depletion, provision of energy requirements, maintenance of the body's defences, and managing fluid and electrolyte balance. Careful attention to nutritional provision should reduce morbidity and mortality.

Critically ill patients present nutritional challenges as a consequence of their pre-existing ill-health, their critical illness and its management. Many are chronically undernourished on admission: causes include alcohol and drug abuse, poor social circumstances, abdominal malignancy, inflammatory bowel disease and chronic cardiac or lung disease. Previously healthy patients may have suffered days of poor oral intake secondary to an acute illness prior to admission to the ICU.

Sepsis and the systemic inflammatory immune response result in increased oxygen consumption and an increase in resting energy expenditure. During critical illness a third of energy demands are met by protein breakdown, leading to significant muscle wasting. Inactivity also contributes to this feature of critical illness, even in adequately fed patients. Gastroparesis and intestinal ileus are very common and result in reduced absorption of feed (Figure 13.1).

Management of critical illness contributes to nutritional deficits: opioids and catecholamines reduce gastric emptying, antibiotics and other drugs cause diarrhoea and sometimes malabsorption, and frequent interruptions to feeding are common. A proactive approach to feeding is essential.

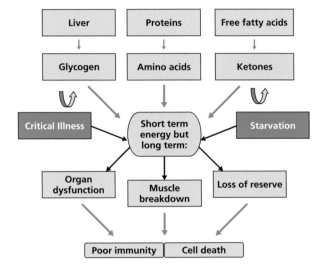

Figure 13.1 Metabolism in the ICU.

Effects of starvation on the gut

In patients already malnourished, lack of enteral feeding leads to mucosal atrophy, loss of integrity of the gut mucosal barrier, increased permeability, decreased absorptive capacity, reduction in gut immunity and loss of cell architecture. In starvation the gut flora are altered, with non-pathogenic species being transformed into pathogenic ones due to a change in their environment. These bacteria may be able to enter the circulation via damaged mucosa and this may contribute to organ damage through a sepsis response. Bacteria may also be aspirated into the lungs past the endotracheal tube and can lead to ventilator-associated pneumonia.

Even if full enteral feed is not tolerated by the gut, a background amount of 10 mL/h may be helpful in preventing these negative effects. Enteral nutrients stimulate gut blood flow, helping to maintain the integrity of cellular architecture and encouraging release of gastrointestinal hormones that regulate the digestion of food.

The refeeding syndrome

This is an under-recognized complication of nutritional support in critical care that can cause considerable morbidity and mortality. Feeding severely malnourished patients initiates a shift from the fatty acid metabolism of starvation back to carbohydrate

ABC of Intensive Care, Second Edition.
Edited by Graham R. Nimmo and Mervyn Singer.
© 2011 Blackwell Publishing Ltd. Published 2011 by Blackwell Publishing Ltd.

Table 13.1 The refeeding syndrome.

Features of refeeding syndrome	Caused by
Cardiac failure, arrhythmias and hypotension Respiratory muscle weakness	Hypophosphataemia, hypomagnesaemia and hypokalaemia
Seizures and neurological damage (e.g. Wernicke's encephalopathy)	Thiamine deficiency and electrolyte derangement (above)
Extracellular fluid expansion: peripheral and pulmonary oedema	Sodium retention due to insulin release
Diarrhoea Immune dysfunction Lactic acidosis	A combination of the above

metabolism with increased phosphate and thiamine requirements, causing acute thiamine deficiency, release of insulin, and an intracellular shift of potassium, magnesium and phosphate. This can result in many adverse effects (Table 13.1). A slow build up of nutrition to full requirements, careful supplementation of phosphate and other electrolytes, thiamine replacement prior to feeding and laboratory monitoring of electrolytes (with appropriate supplementation) can help prevent the disorder. Refeeding syndrome may not present as a clear independent entity but may contribute to the patient's critical illness and pass unrecognized.

Nutritional assessment

It is important to identify malnourished patients in ICU and to assess the risk of refeeding syndrome. The medical history should include height, weight, recent food intake and weight loss. These parameters have been combined in the Malnutrition Universal Screening Tool (MUST) (Box 13.1), which is being widely introduced in the UK and identifies malnourished and 'at-risk' patients. Most critically ill patients fall into the latter category therefore it is important to identify severely malnourished patients who are at risk of refeeding syndrome. Malnourished patients should be fed as soon as possible, preferably within 24 hours of admission and every effort should be made to avoid gaps in feeding. Even well-nourished patients fall into the 'at risk of malnutrition' category when they do not eat for 5 days. Most critically ill patients will be at risk because of their illness and its treatment if they are not fed artificially soon after admission; for these patients feeding is recommended within 48 hours of admission if possible, but the sooner the better.

Box 13.1 **Nutritional assessment**

MUST: Malnourished if any one of the following:

- BMI less than 18.5 kg/m^2
- Unintentional weight loss greater than 10% within the last 3–6 months
- BMI < 20 kg/m^2 and unintentional weight loss >5% within the last 3–6 months

---

At risk of malnutrition if any one of the following:

- Eaten little or nothing for >5 days and/or likely to eat little or nothing for the next 5 days or longer (i.e. most critically ill patients)
- Poor absorptive capacity, and/or high nutrient losses and/or increased nutritional needs from causes such as catabolism (i.e. most critically ill patients)

Patients at risk of developing refeeding syndrome (from NICE guidelines)

- Any ICU patient with one of the following:
  - BMI <16 kg/m^2
  - Unintentional weight loss greater than 15% within the last 3–6 months
  - Little or no nutritional intake for more than 10 days
  - Critically low levels of potassium (<2.5 mmol/L, phosphate <0.32 mmol/L or magnesium <0.5 mmol/L) prior to feeding

  OR any patient with two or more of the following:
  - BMI less than 18.5 kg/m^2
  - Unintentional weight loss greater than 10% within the last 3–6 months
  - Little or no nutritional intake for more than 5 days
  - A history of alcohol excess or chemotherapy

Calculating nutritional requirements in critically ill patients

The NICE Guidelines for Nutrition Support in Adults recommend that the nutritional prescription for patients established on feeding regimens should provide all of the following (Box 13.2), although more exact calculations are made by the dietitian.

Box 13.2 **Basic nutritional requirements (NICE Guidelines)**

Basic nutritional requirements

- 25–35 kcal/kg/day total energy
- 0.8–1.5 g protein (0.13–0.24 g nitrogen)/kg/day
- 30–35 mL fluid/kg/24 h (basic maintenance requirement, including feed, drugs and infusions). Replace losses (drains, bleeding, diarrhoea, gastric losses, fistulae)

Adequate electrolytes, minerals and micronutrients (allowing for deficits, excessive losses or increased demands)

- Add 2.5 mL/kg/24 hours for each degree of temperature above 37°C

A dietitian is an essential member of the multidisciplinary team in the ICU and is responsible for calculating the patient's requirements and prescribing appropriate types of feed (Box 13.3). An attempt is made to account for their metabolic rate and severity of illness. The 'gold standard' of measurement of energy expenditure is indirect calorimetry but this is impractical in most clinical settings. The

Schofield equation is widely used to calculate basal metabolic rate (e.g. for a female >60 years, BMR = $(9.2\times$ weight in kg) + 687 = kcal/day). Adjustments to this figure are made for stress and activity, leading to a figure for total energy expenditure in kcal/day, which is the prescribed calorific requirement.

Box 13.3 **Types of feed**

Types of feed – choose according to needs of individual patients:

- Standard: 1–1.2 kcal/mL, 4–5.55 g protein/100 mL
- High energy: 1.5–2 kcal/mL
- High energy and protein: 2 kcal/mL, 7–8.4 g protein/100 mL
- Low sodium: for hypernatraemic patients
- Low electrolyte and High energy: for patients with renal failure
- Peptide/semi-elemental: for malabsorption/pancreatitis
- Fibre-containing feeds: variable effect on diarrhoea

Many small trials have shown some benefits associated with feeds containing immunonutrients i.e. certain amino acids, anti-oxidants and omega-3 fatty acids. The exact place of these nutrients in parenteral and enteral nutrition in ICU remains to be conclusively established. (Figure 13.2).

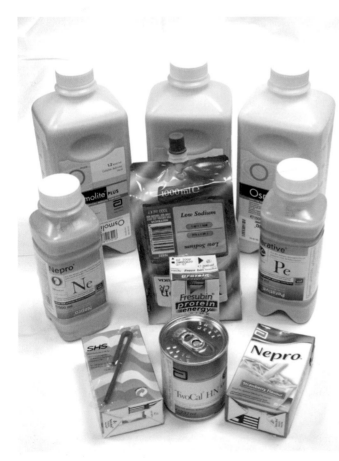

Figure 13.2 Feed bottles.

Routes of feeding

Enteral feeding

This is the delivery of feed via a tube into the stomach, duodenum or jejunum for patients with an accessible gastrointestinal tract who cannot ingest oral feed, or cannot meet demands orally (Figure 13.3). Post-pyloric (duodenal or jejunal) feeding can be considered when there is gastroparesis but a working bowel, or the nasogastric route is inaccessible. Percutaneous endoscopic gastrostomy (PEG) or a radiologically inserted gastrostomy (RIG) can be considered in patients likely to need long-term enteral feeding.

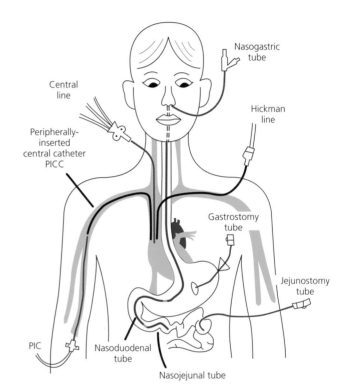

Figure 13.3 Routes of feeding.

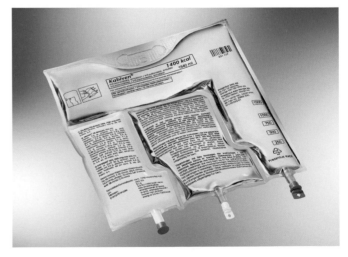

Figure 13.4 Parenteral nutrition bag.

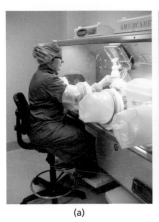
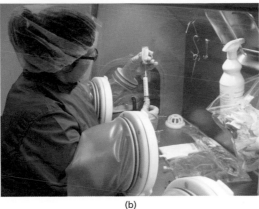
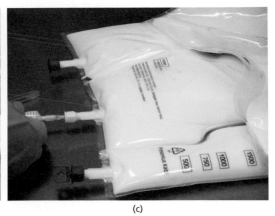

(a)   (b)   (c)

Figure 13.5 (a) A pharmacist prepares the additions to a three-chamber bag of parenteral nutrition in an aseptic manner. (b) A water-soluble vitamin solution is mixed aseptically. (c) The vitamins are introduced into the bag of parenteral nutrition, the partitions of which have now been broken to mix the three chambers.

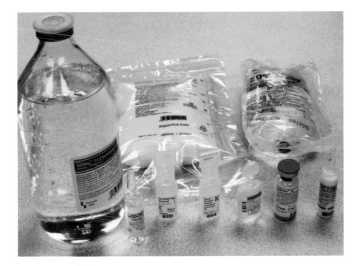

Figure 13.6 The basic ingredients that form parenteral nutrition. From left to right, back row: Amino acids (large glass bottle) fat, glucose; front row: calcium, potassium ×2, trace elements, water-soluble vitamins, fat-soluble vitamins.

Parenteral nutrition

Intravenous nutrition is required in patients who have a non-functional or inaccessible gastrointestinal tract, or who have fistulae. Giving PN to a patient with a functioning gut confers no advantage unless the patient cannot be fed adequately by the enteral route. Guidelines suggest that supplemental PN can be added to meet requirements within 72 hours, or earlier in malnourished patients (Figure 13.4).

A dedicated central catheter lumen is required. Peripheral PN may be given via a peripherally inserted catheter (PIC line). A low osmolality formula is required for this route of access.

PN bags are presented in a three-chambered form to maintain stability of the ingredients and are prescribed according to the patient's blood results and calorific requirements (Figure 13.5). The seals between the chambers are broken before administration to the patient. The pharmacist has a crucial role to play in the preparation of PN (Figure 13.6).

Table 13.2 Complications of feeding.

Enteral feeding	Parenteral feeding
Blockage of tube	Complications related to central venous catheter insertion (bleeding, pneumothorax, vessel damage)
Patient discomfort	Catheter-related bloodstream infection
Skin and mucosal damage	Deranged liver function tests, cholestasis
Inadequate feeding due to interruptions	Gut atrophy if no enteral feed given.
Aspiration of feed into lung causing pneumonia	Overfeeding (uncommon) hyperglycaemia, hyperuricaemia increased triglycerides, fatty liver
Displacement of tube: feeding into lung	
Intolerance – diarrhoea, vomiting	
Gastroparesis: optimize absorption with prokinetics (e.g. metoclopramide, erythromycin)	

Enteral nutrition and PN are not without risk but, if carefully managed by the intensive care team, these risks can be minimized (Table 13.2).

Further reading

Heyland DK, Dhaliwal R, Drover JW, *et al*. Canadian Critical Care Clinical Practice Guidelines Committee. Canadian clinical practice guidelines for nutrition support in mechanically ventilated, critically ill adult patients. *J Parenter Enteral Nutr* 2003; 27: 355–73.

Powell-Tuck, J. *Nutritional interventions in critical illness: Proc Nutrition Soc* 2007; 66: 16–24.

Malnutrition Universal Screening Tool: the Malnutrition Advisory Group of BAPEN 2003 ISBN 1 899467 90 4.

NICE Guidelines: CG032 National Collaborating Centre for Acute Care, February 2006. CG32 Nutrition Support in Adults ISBN 0-9549760-2-9. Oral nutrition support, enteral tube feeding and parenteral nutrition. Guide to Clinical Nutrition. British Dietetic Association.

Online tutorial

There is an online tutorial on this subject at http://www.scottish intensive-care.org.uk/education/index.htm. Click on the 'Induction tutorials' tab to find it.

CHAPTER 14

Critical Care Outreach

Mandy Odell[1] and Sheila Adam[2]

[1]The Royal Berkshire NHS Foundation Trust, Reading, UK
[2]University College, London Hospitals, NHS Foundation Trust, London, UK

> ## OVERVIEW
> The aims of critical care outreach are:
>
> - to improve recognition and management of acutely ill patients in hospital by enhancing acute care knowledge and abilities among ward staff, and supporting interventions in acute/peri-arrest situations
> - to prevent unnecessary admissions to critical care
> - to support discharge from critical care

For many years it has been apparent to intensive care clinicians that earlier recognition of deterioration in hospital inpatients and more rapid referral to intensive care could improve survival. Acute deterioration can be recognized by changes in commonly monitored physiological variables including respiratory rate, blood pressure, heart rate, oxygen saturation and conscious level. An increase in respiratory rate is the most sensitive and often the earliest change in the majority of deteriorating patients but is least well recognized or documented. A number of papers have highlighted the issue of delayed recognition and the following solutions have been proposed:

1 sharing of critical care skills with ward staff
2 introduction of systems that would ensure earlier recognition of deterioration
3 methods of ensuring a skilled response appropriate to the patient's level of need.

Recommendations from the Department of Health resulted in a policy change in England and Wales accompanied by significant funding allowing the set up of critical care outreach services in a large number of acute hospitals. The aim of this initiative was to improve patient care as outlined in the aims stated above. However, a lack of central direction resulted in individual hospitals evolving their own critical care outreach system according to local circumstances. In similar earlier initiatives, medical emergency response teams (MET) had been set up in Australia and the USA, based on the pioneering work of the MET team established in 1990 in Liverpool, Australia.

These teams have all developed acute recognition systems based on the use of commonly monitored physiological variables. Responses to these 'track and trigger' systems vary according to the severity of physiological derangement, ranging from immediate emergency team attendance to an increased frequency of monitoring and early medical staff review.

Track and trigger systems

The aim of such systems is to trigger a clinical response for each individual patient that is neither so specific that it is too late to intervene effectively (e.g. cardiac arrest), nor so sensitive that almost every unwell patient will trigger a call. Sensitivity reflects how good the system is at detecting deteriorating patients, whereas specificity reflects how good it is at excluding patients who are not deteriorating.

There are three types of systems: (1) single-parameter systems characterized by the MET, use any single criterion meeting a specified level of abnormality to trigger a call to the team(Lee *et al.* 1995), (2) multiparameter scoring systems that trigger a referral when one or more criterion is breached and (3) aggregated scoring systems that consist of a number of weighted physiological ranges that are added together for a final score. None of these systems removes the need for direct patient observation and assessment, that is looking at the general demeanour of the patient closely but they empower and initiate the necessary response/call. A small group of patients will be profoundly unwell but may not initially trigger and it may only be through this critical clinical observation that this is recognized. Equally, a small group of patients might trigger who may not be profoundly unwell (e.g. the very fit athlete with low heart rate and blood pressure). An early warning score (EWS) and direct clinical observation are therefore complementary.

Physiological parameters

Risk parameters have been identified from several large studies that looked at physiological derangement associated with serious events such as death, cardiac arrest and emergency admission to intensive care. These include (1) airway compromise, (2) increased respiratory rate, (3) hypotension and (4) a reduced Glasgow Coma Score (GCS). Other monitored variables that showed a less direct association include heart rate changes and falls in urine output.

ABC of Intensive Care, Second Edition.
Edited by Graham R. Nimmo and Mervyn Singer.
© 2011 Blackwell Publishing Ltd. Published 2011 by Blackwell Publishing Ltd.

Table 14.1 An example of an aggregated early warning score system.*

Score	3	2	1	0	1	2	3
Respiratory rate (breaths/min)		≤8		9–14	15–20	21–29	≥30
Heart rate (beats/min)		≤40	41–50	51–100	101–110	111–129	≥130
Blood pressure Systolic, mmHg	≤70	71–80	81–100	101–199		≥200	
Conscious level	Non–responsive	Pain	Voice	Alert			
Urine output (per hour for 2 h)	0	<30	30–44	≥45			

*Trigger level is commonly a score of 3 or 4.

Aggregated scoring systems

With this approach, a risk score is based on accrued abnormal monitored variables, with a set trigger point for intervention. Morgan *et al.* (1997) developed the first EWS, variations of which are commonly used to identify patients who are either at risk of deterioration, or who are clearly deteriorating and in need of increased levels of care. EWS systems can be used with or without an accompanying critical care referral team, although they are more likely to be effective when used together.

The EWS provides a framework for ward staff to guide their response to a deteriorating patient and so can be a useful communication tool usable by staff of all levels of expertise and experience.

The aggregated EWS (Table 14.1) consists of a number of physiological measures with predetermined weighted ranges. Normal values score 0, whereas scores ranging from 1–3 are based on increasing abnormality. When a trigger score is reached, clinical intervention is mandated, for example referral to the Outreach team or to the on-call medical team. The aim of the design and construction of any EWS system is to optimize sensitivity and specificity, while making it as simple as possible for nurses and doctors to use. A balance has to be struck between the sensitivity and specificity of an EWS scoring system and its complexity. A system that has too many items to measure greatly increases the time involved in routine observations, is expensive to implement, or needs high levels of skill and will not be readily applied in practice. As EWSs are developing, more evidence is emerging that highlight the most common and useful parameters for detecting physiological deterioration. Most EWSs include four core components: respiratory rate, pulse rate, systolic blood pressure and conscious level. A recent study evaluating an aggregated scoring system has reported a well-validated EWS that includes six physiological and one interventional element: respiratory rate, heart rate, systolic blood pressure, temperature, conscious level, oxygen saturation and inspired oxygen. Work is in place to develop a national early warning score (NEWS), and it is likely that this will be the benchmark for acute hospitals in the next few years.

Sepsis recognition and response

Early recognition with appropriate support and definitive therapy improves outcomes in the septic patient (Dellinger *et al.* 2008). An important component of critical care outreach is to ensure early recognition of sepsis in ward or emergency department

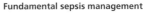

Fundamental sepsis management

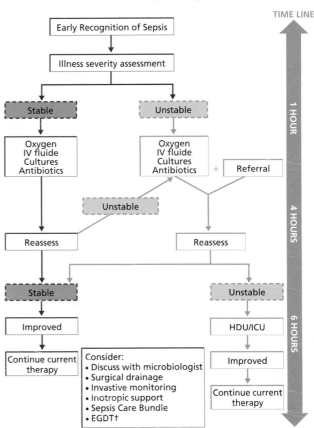

† EGDT - Rivers E, et al: 'Protocol for Early Goal-Directed Therapy'. *N Engl j med* 2001
©Identifying Sepsis Early

Figure 14.1 Early recognition and response for sepsis.

patients, allowing timely resuscitation, investigation, monitoring and antimicrobial therapy. Education of all healthcare staff regarding the early recognition and management of suspected sepsis can make a difference to patient outcomes (www.survivingsepsis.org) (Figure 14.1).

Critical care outreach teams

In the UK these are commonly nurse-led with nurse consultants leading the development of the service. They are drawn from a rota of staff that either provide 24-hour cover (8–10 nurses) or, alternatively, intermittent weekday cover with one or two nurses focusing on education of ward staff and development of acute care skills. These outreach teams support the patient's own medical and nursing teams to deliver an appropriate and effective response to acute deterioration. This response may require urgent involvement of senior intensive care medical staff. In Australia and the USA the MET team is more often multiprofessional, consisting of medical, nursing and other health professionals.

Studies have attempted to prove the efficacy of the outreach concept in improving patient outcomes. Hillman *et al.* (2005) conducted a cluster randomized controlled study in 23 Australian hospitals but could find no significant reduction in unexpected deaths, cardiac arrests or unplanned admission to intensive care following the introduction of METs. This study was however difficult to control (e.g. reporting a lack of recorded observations in patients and non-referrals despite calling criteria being present) and was underpowered statistically. A systematic review of the effectiveness of outreach services undertaken the following year found there was insufficient evidence to conclusively demonstrate improvements in patient outcomes. Nonetheless, outreach systems are firmly established within the English healthcare system, and are recommended as part of a quality care initiative by both the National Patient Safety Agency (2007) and the National Institute for Clinical Excellence (2007).

Ward-based clinical teams greatly value the support offered by outreach teams whose scope of practice has been gradually expanding. Apart from offering support, advice and practical help, they can be instrumental in bringing together different healthcare teams and facilitating optimal care plans for patients and their families, including decisions around the move to palliative care. Skills have also been developed enabling outreach nurses to take arterial blood gases, order investigations and prescribe medication. They may also be part of the cardiac arrest team, have advanced life support skills, and can assist in the care of general ward patients with tracheostomies (Figure 14.2).

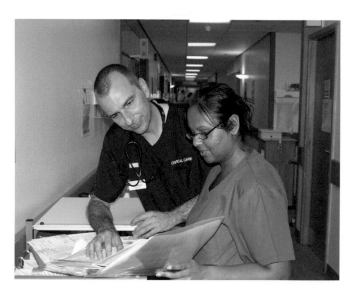

Figure 14.2 An outreach nurse working with a ward nurse.

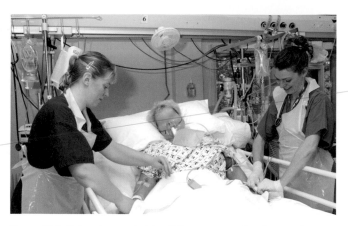

Figure 14.3 Outreach nurse helping ICU prepare a patient for transfer to the ward.

Facilitating discharge from critical care and follow up

The outreach team also work closely with the intensive care unit to ensure that patient discharge is safe and effective. They can be a valuable resource in placing patients in the appropriate clinical area, and in supporting ward staff in their subsequent care. Indeed, critical care outreach has been successful in preventing readmissions to critical care areas and in reducing post-discharge deaths (Figure 14.3).

Patients frequently experience physical and psychological problems post-critical care (Box 14.1). By making sure the patient is physiologically optimized for ward care and psychologically ready and supported, the outreach nurse can reduce the stress of moving between critical care and the ward for both the patient and their family.

Box 14.1 **Common patient problems following critical care**

Common physical problems immediately following critical care

- Recovering organ failure (e.g. lung, kidney, liver etc.)
- Muscle wasting and weakness
  - Reduced cough power
  - Pharyngeal weakness
- Joint pain and stiffness (particularly shoulders)
- Numbness, paraesthesiae (peripheral neuropathy)
- Taste changes (favourite foods become unpalatable)
- Itching, dry skin
- Disturbances of sleep rhythm and pattern
  - Waking at night, poor sleep, not rested
- Cardiac and circulatory decompensation
  - Postural hypotension (autonomic neuropathy)
- Breathlessness on mild exertion
  - Increased work of breathing

Common psychological problems following critical care

- Depression
  - Anger and conflict with the family

- Anxiety
  - About recovery to normal state
  - Panic attacks
  - Fear of dying
- Guilt
- Recurrent nightmares
- Post-traumatic stress disorder

Adapted from Griffiths and Jones (2002).

Critical care outreach supports discharge by:

- improving communication between ward and critical care staff
- educating and supporting ward staff in both general and specific problems facing patients on discharge from critical care
- providing intensive care unit staff with expert advice on the appropriate ward environment and capability for managing specific aspects of the patient's care after ICU discharge, for example tracheostomy care.

The importance of ongoing education and support in the recognition of, and response to, acute deterioration

Even when track and trigger systems are in place, and ward staff have access to expert critical care teams, failure to undertake sufficient vital sign monitoring, to recognize abnormalities or to act according to agreed protocols continue to be an ongoing problem in general hospital wards. Thus, deteriorating patients do not necessarily receive the care they need. In the UK, the National Confidential Enquiry into Patient Outcome and Death study of 439 medical patients admitted to critical care found that only 3.6 sets of observations were recorded on average on the day of admission to critical care. In addition, two-thirds waited more than 12 hours for referral to critical care despite gross physiological abnormalities that were documented and clearly identifiable.

The effectiveness of track and trigger systems and subsequent referral to outreach teams are wholly reliant on ward staff performing timely clinical observation, having a basic understanding of abnormal physiology, and calling promptly for expert help when required.

Education is hugely important in this regard and is one of the biggest impact initiatives offered by critical care outreach. A number of courses (e.g. ALERT, IMPACT, HELP, CCRISP) and freely available web resources (ISE, SICS) are accessible to support education. A strong emphasis is placed on effective communication and multidisciplinary team working in the context of a stressful situation. Enhanced inter-professional understanding, communication and collaboration can impact upon the care of all patients, not just those who become critically ill.

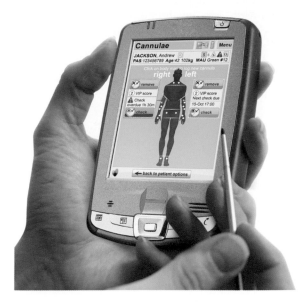

Figure 14.4 Example of electronic charting for ward patients – Vitalpac.

The future

Although significant improvements in patient care have already been made, a number of technological advances may offer considerably better predictive ability for patients at risk of acute deterioration. The advent of electronic charting systems such as Vitalpac™ with inbuilt alert mechanisms and algorithms to prompt correct responses will enhance the ability of staff to provide timely and effective management of acutely deteriorating patients. Additional technology using computerized modelling of multiple physiological variables may also support more accurate prediction of risk allowing preventive interventions. These will not replace the need to assess the patient effectively and to combine electronic information with bedside review. It remains to be seen whether this technology will become a feature of ward care due to the cost (Figure 14.4).

Further reading

Adam S, Odell M and Welch J. *Rapid assessment of the acutely ill patient*. Wiley-Blackwell: Oxford, 2010.

Cioffi J. Nurses' experience of making decisions to call emergency assistance to their patients. *J Adv Nurs* 2000; 32:108–14.

Department of Health. *Comprehensive Critical Care: a review of adult critical care services*. The Stationary Office: London, 2000.

Esmonde L, McDonnell A, Ball C, *et al*. (2006). Investigating the effectiveness of critical care outreach services: a systematic review. *Intensive Care Med* 32:1713–21.

Featherstone P, Smith GB, Linnelld M, *et al*. Impact of a one-day inter-professional course (ALERT™) on attitudes and confidence in managing critically ill adult patients. *Resuscitation* 2005; 65:329–36.

Goldhill DR, Worthington L, Mulcahy A, *et al.* The patient-at-risk team: identifying and managing seriously ill ward patients. *Anaesthesia* 1999; 54:853–60.

Lee, A., G. Bishop, Hillman KM, *et al.* The Medical Emergency Team. *Anaesth Intensive Care* 1995; 23:183–6.

Morgan RJM, Williams F, Wright MM. An early warning system for detecting developing critical illness. *Clin Intensive Care* 1997; 8:100.

NCEPOD. *An Acute Problem?* NCEPOD: London, 2005.

NICE. *The Acutely Ill Patient in Hospital. Centre for Clinical Practice.* NICE: London, 2007.

NPSA. *Safer Care for the Acutely Ill Patient: learning from serious incidents.* NPSA: London, 2007.

Prytherch DR, Smith GB, Schmidt PE, Featherstone PI. ViEWS –towards a national early warning score for detecting adult inpatient deterioration. *Resuscitation* 2010; 81:932–7.

CHAPTER 15

End-of-Life Care

Ben Shippey[1] and Bob Winter[2]

[1]NHS Fife, Fife, Scotland
[2]Queens Medical Centre, Nottingham, UK

OVERVIEW

- End-of-life care is an important core activity in intensive care
- Approximately 20–30% of patients admitted to intensive care will die
- Decisions must often be made regarding the appropriateness of continuation of treatment and support
- Quality of survival must be taken into account
- Conversations about these decisions should be honest and sensitive and should involve the patient and family, if possible
- Advanced directives can help to determine the wishes of the patient lacking competency
- The possibility of organ donation should always be considered

Introduction

Although 20–30% of patients die during their stay in intensive care, it is relatively unusual for this to occur unpredictably. Far more commonly, there is a process of either withholding or withdrawing treatment that ultimately results in death. There is necessarily a point during the patient's admission when a decision is made that either ongoing treatment is futile and will not result in survival (Box 15.1), or that the burden of ongoing treatment outweighs the chances of the patient regaining an acceptable quality of life. At this point there is a realignment of clinical priorities away from 'life support' and specific treatment with the intention of aiding survival, towards a palliative model of care with the intention of providing a dignified, symptom-free death.

Box 15.1 **Futility**

A treatment is futile when it will not achieve the outcome for which it is intended. The definition of the intended outcome is therefore essential when discussing futility. In the context of intensive care, physiological futility can be defined by the failure of a parameter to improve despite intervention, and therapeutic futility as the outcome is that the patient will die despite maximal therapy. Futility is a difficult concept to apply, as it is often difficult to be certain that the intended outcome will not be achieved

When deciding to withhold or withdraw treatment and ongoing life support, the balance of the burden of ongoing treatment must be weighed against the likelihood and predicted quality of survival and its likely acceptability to the patient. Intensive care treatment is unpleasant. Survivors list pain, anxiety, breathlessness, thirst, hunger, inability to speak and hallucinations as causes of distress during their intensive care admission, although they often describe this as a price that was worth paying. Patients and relatives have widely varying expectations of intensive care unit outcome. The survival of intensive care and cardiac arrest patients portrayed in films and television dramas is artificially high, and the patient's return to normal activity often unrealistically rapid and complete. Not all patients return to normal after an intensive care admission. Many experience a prolonged period of complex emotional, psychological and/or physical disturbance that can have a significant impact on their quality of life. Despite this, many are content with the quality of life that they achieve. Clinicians often overestimate the burden of care and underestimate the value placed on survival by patients and their families. Religious affiliation (of healthcare professionals, patients and families) can also affect end of life decisions. For example, Judaism teaches that all life is of equal value and so the concept of 'quality of life' is not relevant to the discussion. As a result, conversations with families about the balance between the burden of treatment and the patient's chances of an acceptable quality of survival can be difficult, with consensus of opinion being difficult to reach.

In an ideal world the decision to withdraw (or withhold) treatment should generally be made in consultation with the patient. However, as this is not often possible in the critically ill patient lacking capacity, clinicians are left to make a decision that they judge to be in the patient's 'best interests' (Box 15.2). Such decisions are made, where possible, in consultation with the patient's family and close friends, who are asked to provide a surrogate

ABC of Intensive Care, Second Edition.
Edited by Graham R. Nimmo and Mervyn Singer.
© 2011 Blackwell Publishing Ltd. Published 2011 by Blackwell Publishing Ltd.

for the patient's wishes for ongoing treatment. It is vitally important that family members do not feel that they are being asked to *make* the decision, or worse, asked for *'permission to turn the life support machine off'*. It is worth stating explicitly during the discussions that *'We are making this decision on behalf of your relative with your input on their likely feelings'*. The practice of including families in end-of-life decision-making may increase their long-term risk of psychological problems, so it is essential that these conversations are handled sensitively to minimize future distress.

Box 15.2 **Best interests**

Prolonging the patient's life is normally in their best interests. The quality of that survival must be weighed against the burden of treatment. If the burden of treatment outweighs the quality of the likely survival it is unlikely that the treatment is in the patients 'best interests'

In patients likely to require intensive care treatment at some stage in the future, such as those with degenerative neurological conditions or advanced chronic respiratory disease, it can be extremely useful to discuss with them the implications of intensive care admission, and to make a prospective decision based on their wishes. Unfortunately, intensive care admission is often unpredictable, and patients are often treated on the basis that they *would* want the care that is offered. However, patients who feel strongly that they would not want intensive care treatment may make an advanced directive, or 'living will'. This allows the patient to decline certain treatments *a priori*, or to appoint a surrogate decision-maker who will make decisions if they become incapacitated to the extent that they are unable to decide for themselves. An advanced directive is only valid if the patient had capacity when they made the decision, were fully informed about the consequences, were not put under pressure and have not subsequently given any indication that they have changed their mind. Although currently uncommon in the UK, such advanced directives can be very helpful when decisions about intensive care treatment have to be made. In England and Wales, an independent mental capacity advocate may be appointed to act on behalf of a patient who lacks capacity and has no family member or individual with lasting power of attorney to represent their wishes.

Once a decision has been made that ongoing life-supporting treatment is either futile or excessively burdensome, the aim of the ICU team should be to provide 'a good death'. The definition of 'a good death' varies, but there are some common themes. When people were asked (in the context of a BBC television documentary) about their wishes for end of life care, being at home with family members and free from pain were rated highly. It is easy to see how these wishes can be forgotten in the highly technological environment of the ICU. Commonly recurring themes from the families of dying intensive care patients are the need for information, explanation and understanding, the need to be with their relative, and the need to be able to express emotion. It should be possible to achieve good symptom control in the intensive

care setting. Staff can find it very rewarding to support a patient and their family through the dying process and the subsequent period.

Withdrawal and withholding treatment

Clinical practice around the withholding and withdrawal of organ support is highly variable, both between intensive care units and between clinicians working in the same intensive care unit. It may be helpful to use a protocol both to ensure consistency and to provide support of, and protection for, staff involved in the withdrawal process. Many strategies are used during treatment withdrawal. Commonly, a combination of weaning of ventilatory support, cessation of renal support, and discontinuation of vasopressor and inotrope infusions is employed. Some clinicians may remove the endotracheal tube or tracheostomy if deemed appropriate to do so. Infusions of sedatives and opioids are used to ease the symptoms of breathlessness, pain and anxiety. The use of muscle relaxants is inappropriate in this situation as they have no use in symptom control unless mandatory ventilation is continued, and may mask symptoms that would otherwise require treatment. Unnecessary treatments such as antibiotics should be discontinued.

From an ethical viewpoint there is no difference between withdrawing and withholding a treatment that is sustaining, or would sustain, life. However, from an emotional standpoint many intensive care clinicians find it easier to withhold a treatment than to withdraw it once it has started. Common limitations to treatment and support include withholding of tracheal intubation, limiting the dose of inotrope or vasopressor, limiting inspired oxygen concentration, or withholding renal replacement therapy. The potential problem with treatment-limiting decisions is confusion over the true intent of therapy. There can be a slow 'fade' of curative treatment intent without a positive decision being made in favour of palliative treatment, and with less emphasis placed on symptom control as a result. Families may find it difficult to understand why some treatments are not being used and this can make ensuing conversations about palliative care more difficult.

Brain death and organ donation

If intracranial pressure rises acutely and to a high level the brainstem can be compressed and become ischaemic or infarcted. Vital structures controlling respiratory and cardiovascular physiology cease to function. Artificial support of cardiovascular and respiratory systems will maintain the body physiologically for a time (possibly days) but cardiac arrest is eventually inevitable. Once brain death has occurred, further organ support is futile, and should ultimately be discontinued. In some patients where organ donation is possible organ support is continued for a short while and death is confirmed by formal brain-stem death testing. Once brain stem death has been diagnosed, and assent from the patient's family has been obtained, organ retrieval can occur. It is also important to identify patients in whom brain death has occurred, but who are not potential donors, in order to prevent futile continuation of organ support.

Rates of organ donation vary widely internationally and across communities, largely as a result of cultural and religious differences in attitude towards transplantation. In the UK, at present, there is no 'presumed consent' to organ donation. Patients (ideally) give consent, or their families give assent, for organ retrieval to take place. There is ongoing discussion about this procedure and the legal framework around organ donation may change in the near future. Just over half of UK families of potential organ donors give their assent to organ retrieval. Checking whether the patient has joined the UK organ donor register can be very helpful at this point. Reasons for withholding assent include knowing that the patient was opposed, being uncertain about the patient's wishes, divided opinion among the relatives, unwillingness to submit the patient to further surgery, and the view that the patient had 'suffered enough'.

The subject of organ donation must be approached sensitively and at an appropriate time (often after the first set of brain death tests). The consultant intensivist caring for the patient usually makes the initial approach to the patient's family, but there is evidence from the USA (where intensive care is organized very differently) that involving a transplant coordinator at an earlier stage in the process may improve the rate of organ donation. This has yet to be proven in the very different environment of the UK, where many consultant intensivists look upon this aspect of patient care as part of their professional responsibility to the patient. If assent for organ donation is given, the patient is transferred to an operating theatre at a convenient time and transplantable organs are removed after confirming suitability and safety. Transplantable organs are increasingly being retrieved immediately after death by cardiac arrest, although organ retrieval after confirmation of brainstem death still remains much more common in the UK.

The process of determination of brain death varies in different countries. In the UK the diagnosis is clinical, and there are certain conditions that must be met (Box 15.3). In other countries, EEG evidence, or cerebral oximetry is required. Brain death testing is performed by two senior doctors, one of whom should be a consultant, who do the tests together. Dr A performs while Dr B observes and then vice versa. The time of death is recorded as the time that the first set of brain death tests are performed: the second set is confirmatory.

Box 15.3 **Brain death testing criteria**

Preconditions (must be met)

- Diagnosis compatible with brainstem death
- Presence of irreversible structural brain damage
- Presence of apnoeic coma

Exclusions (must be absent)

- Therapeutic drug effects (sedatives, hypnotics, muscle relaxants)
- Hypothermia (> 35°C)
- Metabolic abnormalities
- Endocrine abnormalities
- Intoxication

Brainstem reflexes (must be absent)

- No pupillary response to light
- Absent corneal reflex
- No motor response within cranial nerve distribution
- Absent gag reflex
- Absent cough reflex
- Absent vestibulo-ocular reflex

Persistent apnoea (must be present)

Further reading

Academy of Royal Colleges, 2008. A code of practice for the diagnosis and confirmation of death. www.breakingbadnews.co.uk – an industry supported site with helpful guidance on end-of-life conversations.

English V. *Withholding and withdrawing life prolonging treatment*. BMA, Supplement to Critical Care Medicine February 2001, Vol 29, Issue 2.

GMC. *Withholding and withdrawing life-prolonging treatments: good practice in decision-making*. London: General Medical Council. http://www.gmc-uk.org/guidance/current/library/witholding_lifeprolonging_guidance.asp.

Saxon R. *Critical Care Focus – Ethical Issues in Intensive Care*. Intensive Care Society.

SUPPORT Principal Investigators 'A controlled trial to improve care for seriously ill hospitalised patients; The Study to Understand Prognoses and Preferences for Outcomes and Risks of Treatment (SUPPORT)' *JAMA* 1995; 274:1591–98.

Index